W0091418

Hydrocephalus

VOLUME 3: CONCEPTS IN NEUROSURGERY

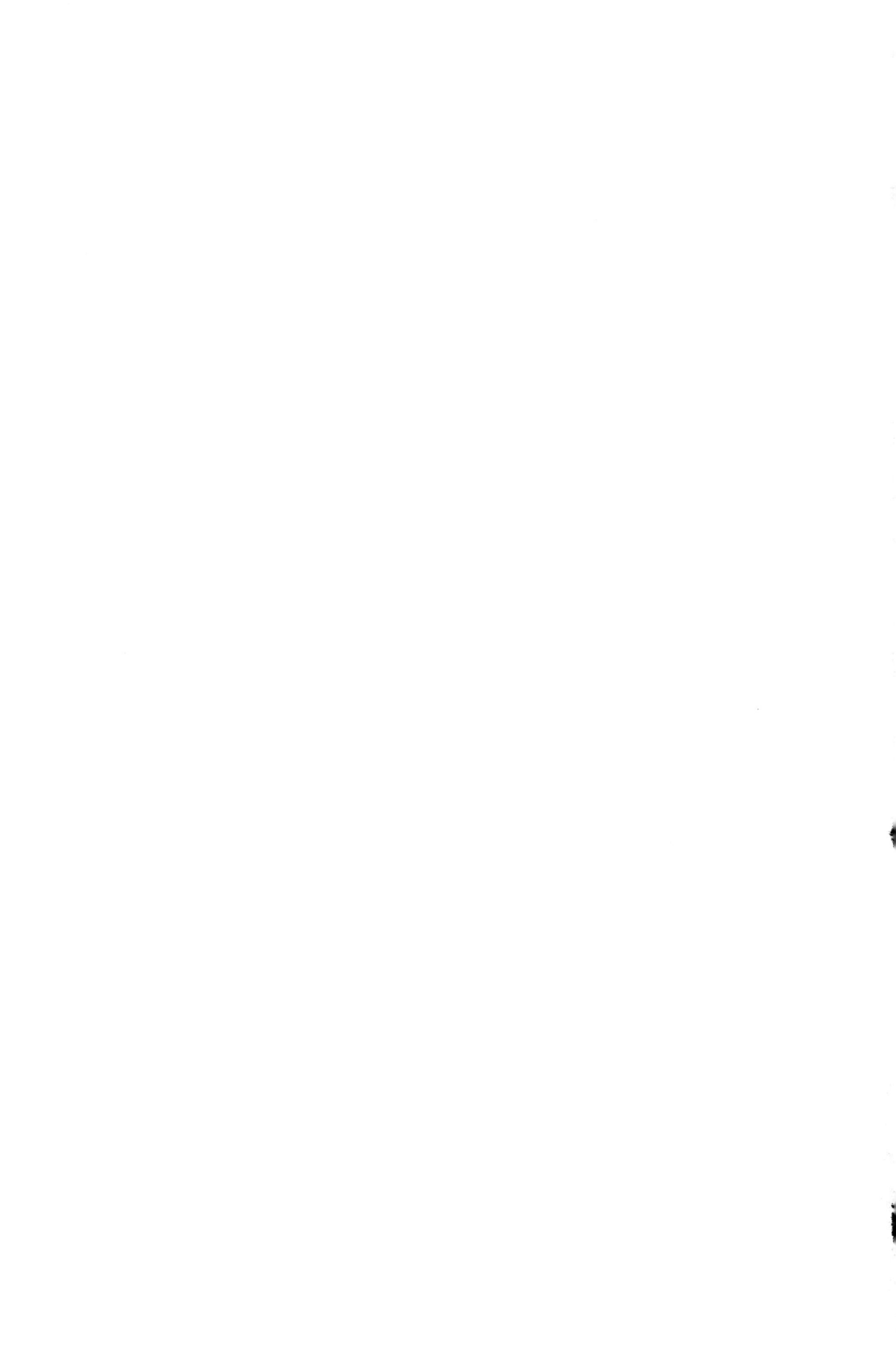

Series Foreword

The Congress of Neurological Surgeons was founded in 1951 with the prime purposes being to maintain high standards of neurosurgery and to promote continuing education. While the emphasis has been on the needs of the resident in training and the younger neurosurgeon, the programs of the Congress have benefited not only neurosurgery but also the neuroscience fields in general.

To help provide for the continuing education needs of its members, the Congress began publication in 1953 of an annual volume entitled *Clinical Neurosurgery*, which presents in detail the invited presentations made at the annual meeting of the organization. This volume has become an important reference source for neurosurgeons. Then in 1977, after several years of planning, the Congress began publication of a monthly journal entitled *Neurosurgery*, which proved to be an outstanding addition to the medical literature.

Now, under the direction of Doctors Fremont P. Wirth and Robert A. Ratcheson, the Congress is embarking on another publication series entitled *Concepts in Neurosurgery*. The goals of this publication, as proposed by Dr. Ratcheson during his term as President of the Congress, are to provide a monograph that will cover a specific area in depth with basic scientific knowledge and theory applied to practical neurosurgical issues. For the resident in training this publication can supplement the educational program or provide knowledge in an area that might not be covered in depth in a training program. For the trained neurosurgeon, each monograph will provide the opportunity to review recent knowledge about a practical subject and supply up-to-date information in an important area of neurosurgery.

The Congress has selected Doctors Wirth and Ratcheson as editors, two individuals who have been members of the Executive Committee for several years and have recently been officers, who have also had considerable experience with educational programs. They will be aided by associate editors, Doctors Robert L. Grubb, Julian T. Hoff, and Martin Weiss, who also have had broad experience with publications and continuing education endeavors.

The Congress is again providing a leadership role in an important area that will benefit all of neurosurgery.

Robert G. Ojemann, M.D.

Foreword

This is the third volume in the series *Concepts in Neurosurgery* and represents the commitment of the Congress of Neurological Surgeons to continuing education in neurosurgery. The editor, R. Michael Scott, has carefully organized this book to address the many facets of hydrocephalus. A distinguished group of authors has been selected because of their expertise in such areas as cerebrospinal fluid physiology, modern imaging, therapeutic techniques, the management of hydrocephalus, and the complications of its treatment.

This monograph fulfills well the aims of *Concepts in Neurosurgery*. It will provide neurosurgeons in training and in practice with up-to-date concepts and promises to serve as a valuable resource in this field. The publication of this volume by the Congress of Neurological Surgeons is expected to enhance the field of neurosurgery and improve the care of our patients.

Fremont P. Wirth, M.D., F.A.C.S.
Robert A. Ratcheson, M.D., F.A.C.S.

Preface

Hydrocephalus is a common neurosurgical problem. Neurosurgeons understand its basic pathophysiology and carry out surgical procedures to treat it. Nevertheless, experienced neurosurgeons realize that the treatment of hydrocephalus is deceptively simple and that a poorly conceived and executed shunt procedure, for example, can have ramifications that affect a patient for the rest of his/her life. We who treat and follow patients with this condition are well aware that there is much to be learned about our therapeutic techniques and their sequelae.

This monograph is our attempt to assemble in one place current concepts in the theory, diagnosis and treatment of hydrocephalus. The contributors were chosen because of their acknowledged expertise in specific areas, and I have been fortunate in having a close personal and professional association with many of them. David McCullough has written previously on the history and treatment of hydrocephalus and is the author of numerous papers regarding its present day management. Harold Rekate is well known for his laboratory, mathematical, and clinical studies of intraventricular CSF dynamics and flow. Samuel Wolpert, my former colleague at the New England Medical Center, has written extensively on the radiologic diagnosis of hydrocephalus and its causes throughout the development of pneumoencephalography, angiography, CT, and MRI. Herbert Gilmore, also a former colleague at the New England Medical Center, has devoted much of his clinical and laboratory research work to the nonsurgical treatment of hydrocephalus. J. Gordon McComb, a recognized authority in pediatric neurosurgery, directs a service where hundreds of shunt procedures are carried out every year. Arthur Marlin is well-known for his work on the treatment of hydrocephalus following intraventricular hemorrhage in premature infants. Jeffrey Wisoff and Fred Epstein are professional colleagues at an active referral center for difficult pediatric neurosurgical problems; Epstein's contributions to the treatment of hydrocephalus and slit ventricle syndrome span several decades. David Klein has written extensively on hydrocephalus and related topics. Michael Edwards and Roger Hudgins practice at an institution that has pioneered the intrauterine diagnosis and treatment of hydrocephalus. Peter Black has been a frequent contributor to the literature on treatment of normal pressure hydrocephalus in adults.

I am grateful to each of the authors for their contributions to this volume, and to Phil Wirth for entrusting me with the task of editing it. I owe special thanks to my family and friends for their patience and support.

R. Michael Scott, M.D.

Contributors

SERIES EDITORS

Fremont P. Wirth, M.D.
Neurological Institute of Savannah
Director, Neurosurgical and Neurological
  Intensive Care Unit
St. Joseph's Hospital
Savannah, Georgia

Robert A. Ratcheson, M.D.
Professor and Chief
  Division of Neurological Surgery
Case Western Reserve University
University Hospitals of Cleveland
Cleveland, Ohio

SERIES ASSOCIATE EDITORS

Robert L. Grubb, Jr., M.D.
Professor of Neurological Surgery
Washington University School of Medicine
St. Louis, Missouri

Julian T. Hoff, M.D.
Professor of Surgery
Head, Section of Neurosurgery
University of Michigan Hospital
Ann Arbor, Michigan

Martin H. Weiss, M.D.
Professor and Chairman
Department of Neurosurgery
LAC/USC Medical Center
Los Angeles, California

VOLUME EDITOR

R. Michael Scott, M.D.
Director, Section of Pediatric Neurosurgery
The Children's Hospital
Associate Professor of Surgery
Harvard Medical School
Boston, Massachusetts

CONTRIBUTORS

Peter McL. Black, M.D., Ph.D.
The Franc D. Ingraham Professor of
  Neurosurgery
Harvard Medical School
Neurosurgeon-in-Chief
Brigham and Women's Hospital and
  The Children's Hospital
Boston, Massachusetts

Michael S. B. Edwards, M.D.
Director, Division of Pediatric Neurosurgery
Professor of Neurosurgery and Pediatrics
Department of Neurological Surgery
University of California School of Medicine
San Francisco, California

Fred J. Epstein, M.D.
Assistant Professor
   Division of Pediatric Neurosurgery
New York University Medical Center
New York, New York

Sarah J. Gaskill, M.D.
Division of Neurosurgery
Duke University Medical Center
Durham, North Carolina

Herbert E. Gilmore, M.D.
Assistant Professor of Pediatrics
Tufts University School of Medicine
Boston, Massachusetts
Division of Pediatric Neurology
Department of Pediatrics
Baystate Medical Center
Springfield, Massachusetts

Roger J. Hudgins, M.D.
Attending Pediatric Neurosurgeon
Scottish Rite Children's Hospital
Atlanta, Georgia

David M. Klein, M.D.
Associate Professor of Neurosurgery
State University of New York at Buffalo
   School of Medicine
Chief, Department of Neurosurgery
Children's Hospital of Buffalo
Buffalo, New York

Arthur E. Marlin, M.D.
Clinical Associate Professor of Pediatrics and
   Orthopedics
University of Texas Health Science Center at
   San Antonio
Head, Section of Pediatric Neurosurgery
Santa Rosa Children's Hospital
San Antonio, Texas

J. Gordon McComb, M.D.
Professor and Head, Division of Neurosurgery
Children's Hospital of Los Angeles
Department of Neurological Surgery
University of Southern California School of
   Medicine
Los Angeles, California

David C. McCullough, M.D.
Chairman, Department of Neurosurgery
Children's Hospital National Medical Center
Professor of Neurological Surgery
George Washington University
Washington, D.C.

William Olivero, M.D.
Section of Pediatric Neurosurgery
Barrow Neurological Institute
Phoenix, Arizona

Harold Rekate, M.D.
Chief, Section of Pediatric Neurosurgery
Barrow Neurological Institute
Phoenix, Arizona

R. Michael Scott, M.D.
Director, Section of Pediatric Neurosurgery
The Children's Hospital
Associate Professor of Surgery
Harvard Medical School
Boston, Massachusetts

Jeffrey H. Wisoff, M.D.
Professor and Director
   Division of Pediatric Neurosurgery
New York University Medical Center
New York, New York

Samuel M. Wolpert, M.D.
Professor of Radiology and Neurology
Tufts University School of Medicine
Chief, Section of Neuroradiology
Department of Radiology
New England Medical Center
Boston, Massachusetts

Contents

CHAPTER 1

History of the Treatment of Hydrocephalus

DAVID C. MCCULLOUGH, M.D.

INTRODUCTION

"Hardly any other pathologic condition has been accorded more determined attention on the part of the medical profession with the aim of finding a cure for it than hydrocephalus. And in hardly a single other condition have cures been so illusive or so often wrecked on purely mechanical obstacles."

Leo M. Davidoff, 1929

A review of the chronology of the treatment of hydrocephalus reaffirms the familiar relationship between basic science and therapeutics. Davidoff's comment (26) in his exhaustive 1929 treatise on the history of the treatment of hydrocephalus is nearly as appropriate today as it was at the time of his writing. Presciently, he appended the opinion, "Yet the outlook is not hopeless." Even though outstanding developments in controlling this condition have evolved since the middle 1950's, cure remains elusive. Neurosurgeons may still find control of the condition "wrecked on purely mechanical obstacles," even in our era of rather routine diagnosis and standard therapy of hydrocephalus. Clinicians can look to Davidoff's statement for inspiration and stimulus to improve approaches and techniques.

Although hydrocephalus was a condition recognized by ancient care-givers and Hippocrates has been acknowledged repeatedly as an early therapist, the evidence for this citation is apparently suspect (26). Anecdotal accounts of diagnosing and treating the disorder from the pre-Christian era were part of a sustained and vague gestational period of therapeutic endeavors that extended into the 20th century. Retrospective examination of the record discloses three rather distinct developmental periods (73): the first circumscribes the dawn of history until the late 19th century; the second or early

scientific period spanned about six decades, and concluded in the third or present epoch, which is characterized by engineering approaches with more or less standard techniques for managing the condition. The student of this record will find several very useful historical accounts, including the fascinating and sobering writings of Haynes (47), Davidoff (26), Scarff (103), Pudenz (95), Milhorat (77), and Wallman (116).

ELEMENTS OF HYDROCEPHALUS

Recognition of the pathophysiology and potential therapy of any disorder requires basic anatomical and physiological data. Early commentators apparently did not precisely understand the location of the abnormal fluid collection within the cranium (51), and hydrocephalus was often confused with subdural effusions. The foundation for modern understanding of the structure of the cerebral ventricles and their role in containing fluid was a product of the 18th century (15) (77). Anatomical writings of the 1760's described the structure of the ventricles and the character of the cerebrospinal fluid (CSF) (15), and during the same decade Morgagne (79) and Whytt (119) provided initial descriptions of the pathology of hydrocephalus. The 19th century investigators, including Magendie (67) and Luschka (77), introduced the concept of CSF circulation. In 1875 Key and Retzius (61) pioneered documentation of ventricular and CSF pathways. Fresh therapeutic approaches for hydrocephalus followed upon those basic descriptions. Early in the 20th century the physiological investigations of Weed (117), Dandy and Blackfan (21), and others probably stimulated the growing therapeutic interest of clinicians. Although the intricacies of the CSF circulation are still incompletely understood, substantial contributions from many laboratories over several decades have paralleled modern therapeutic efforts (10, 20, 27, 87, 117).

The mysteries of the anatomy of hydrocephalus proved difficult to solve. Diagnostic accounts and brief descriptions cited by Whytt in his engaging *Observations on the Dropsy in the Brain* reveal that the ancients were not altogether certain of the location of the excess fluid within the brain (119). Several authors of the 13th and 16th centuries postulated the occurrence of hydrocephalus or described its existence (11, 51, 19). Whytt's lucid descriptions of morbidly declining hydrocephalic patients are difficult to reconcile with our experience in physical diagnosis. Typical of the accounts of that day, description of cutaneous signs, behavioral changes, and vital signs predominated, a striking contrast with the sparse physical examination data and extensive radiographic information characteristic of modern reports.

The relatively recent introduction of ventriculography by Dandy (22) in 1918 was probably the single most important stimulus of therapeutic advance for hydrocephalus. Computerized tomography (CT), magnetic resonance imaging (MRI), and the refinement of ultrasonic imaging in the past two decades have finally brought us to an era of prenatal disclosure of hydrocephalus, introducing the prospect of the fetus as a neurosurgical patient.

THE FIRST ERA: PRIMITIVE EFFORTS

The first era in the treatment of hydrocephalus from the dawn of history to late in the 19th century entailed as much observation as it did intervention. Unsubstantiated accounts credit Hippocrates with first puncturing dilated ventricles through the open fontanelle or after trephination. Whytt's advice that ". . . in a dropsy of the ventricles of the brain, any such attempt to draw off the water could have no other effect than to hasten death," (119) must have been intimidating to even the most ambitious clinicians. For treatment, as Davidoff (26) relates, patients were "purged, puked, and bled."

Whytt suggested treating hydrocephalus with purgatives, diuretics, blisters, frictions, exercise and diet. Rhubarb, jalop, and calomel as well as oil of asarum were the popular purga-

TABLE 1.1.

Stages in the Pharmacological Therapy of Hydrocephalus.

Era	Drug	Category or Purpose
Antiquity (119)	"Volatile oil"	?
	Cinnamon water	Astringent
	Jalap	Purgative
	Rhubarb	Purgative
	Calomel	Purgative
	Wine	? Sedative
	Asarum	Purgative
Early Scientific (26, 30, 40, 44)	Antipyrene	Antiinflammatory
	Potassium bromide	Diuretic
	Potassium iodide	Diuretic
	Salicylates	Antiinflammatory
	Thyroid extract	Choroid inhibition
Modern (73, 77, 106, 118, 119)	Thyroid extract	Choroid inhibition
	Vital dyes	Choroid inhibition
	Hypertonic sucrose	Diuretic
	Acetazolamide	Diuretic
	Isosorbide	Diuretic
	Glycerol	Diuretic
	Furosamide	Diuretic
	Adrenal corticosteroids	Antinflammatory

tives of the day (119). Success was not expected, as evidenced by Whytt's admission, "I freely own that I have never been so lucky as to cure one patient who had those symptoms which with certainty denoted this disease, and I suspect that those who imagine they have been more successful have mistaken another distemper for this." Table 1.1 lists the medications and their categories as prescribed by the ancients and progressing up to the modern day. Mercury, potassium, iodine, salicylates, and bromines as well oral cinnamon water were common "physics" of the early era (26, 119).

Head binding (12) was another ancient technique obviously recommending itself as clinicians observed progressive head expansion in infants. Interestingly, this method was revived recently by Epstein and his colleagues (33), whose enthusiasm was based on laboratory experiments that supported the ancient empiricists.

As late as 1843, leeching or blood-letting was recommended for acute inflammatory forms of hydrocephalus and "cupping in the vicinity of the mastoid" was advocated for the chronic forms (9). Physical methods included tight binding (12), injection of strong iodine solutions in the ventricles (12), and exposure to the sun, the latter advocated by several 19th-century authors (26, 110). Davidoff later commented that "roentgen rays have at the present time eclipsed the sun in this connection," citing early 20th-century sources (104, 107).

Various surgical approaches of the preantiseptic era included ventricular punctures via fontanelles, cranial sutures, nose, and orbit, and skull trephination. Carotid artery ligation was recommended as early as 1796 (26), and applied sporadically up through the early 20th century (39).

Sparse data exist to help us evaluate these earnest efforts. One must assure that cures were exceptional and complications ubiquitous.

THE SECOND ERA: SURGICAL INITIATIVES

For practical purposes the only dependable therapy for progressive hydrocephalus has been surgery. Although the ideal therapy would be the removal of a known block in the CSF pathways, permanent CSF bypass procedures or some method to reduce CSF production could suffice to control the condition. Since the advent of neurological surgery later in the 19th century, the removal of intracranial mass lesions such as tumors and developmental cysts has produced cures in limited numbers of selected patients. Concomitant with the attempt to cure the condition has been the development of many ingenious procedures to divert the CSF to effective absorptive sites.

Lumbar puncture (LP), first described by Quincke in 1891 as a treatment for hydrocephalus (97), survives today not only as a diagnostic procedure but as a temporary measure for the management of communicating hydrocephalus (43). Carotid artery ligation was recommended by Fraser and Dott (39), who reported encouraging results in three out of four patients in 1922. Fuller (41) in 1927 reported a single successful case attributed to a refined technique.

Although ventricular puncture was nearly always followed by death in the 18th century, single punctures as well as continuous external ventricular drainage occasionally succeeded in the antiseptic era. Keen (58) and others (14) are credited with either suggesting or performing continuous ventricular drainage. According to Davidoff (26), "In spite of antiseptic and aseptic precautions patients died of infection, intercurrent disease, rapid release of intracranial pressure and no demonstrable reason."

Diversion of ventricular or extraventricular fluid to likely internal absorptive sites has captured the interest of many surgeons since the 1890's. Miculicz first attempted drainage to the subcutaneous (subgaleal) space from the lateral ventricle (75) with a "nail" of glass wool, resulting in resolution of the hydrocephalus. He and others later used gold tubes with flanged discs positioned distally in the subgaleal space over the skull. Gold tubes and catgut strands as well as rubber tubes were also used although in limited numbers of cases with indifferent results, and glass tubes, coiled silver wires, silver tubes, linen threads, and omental strips also served as conduits (5) (26, 62, 105) from the ventricle to subgaleal, subdural, or subarachnoid spaces. A report by Sharpe (105) in 1917 disclosed that among 41 cases treated with linen threads (from the ventricle in noncommunicating hydrocephalus and subarachnoid spaces in communicating hydrocephalus), 13 patients died within 36 hours and in 5 there was no improvement; however, 23 improved and 5 were said to have had "remarkable" benefit.

Puncture of the corpus callosum with drainage to the subdural space was introduced by Anton and von Bramann (6, 13) in 1908. This was called the "Balkenstich method." Operative mortality was high and cures were infrequent (28). Internal drainage by lysis of adhesions in the posterior fossa was attempted without success around the turn of the century by Parkin (88), and by Glynn and Thomas (42) with control of hydrocephalus. Murphy (80) and Dandy (24) used this method with some success around 1901 and 1921, respectively. Small numbers of patients were also subjected to aqueductal cannulation (23, 39). Drainage via the orbital roof (ventriculo-orbitotomy) was described by Hildenbrand in 1923 (52). That author noted that "one patient improved for a time." Sokolowski and Irger (109) used Hildenbrand's procedure in six cases, failing each time. Their alternative method of draining the temporal horn of the ventricle to the fatty tissue of the cheek via subtemporal craniectomy was only marginally superior.

Drainage to the vascular system was pioneered by Payr in 1908 using autologous or homologous donor veins to the sagittal sinus and later to the jugular (90). Subsequently, Payr employed hardened calves' arteries within venous sheaths with some success (91), but his results could not be duplicated until the development of fabricated plastic tubes with unidirectional valves in the 1950's. An intriguing autogenous tibial artery bypass from ventricle to superficial temporal vein was also reported by Enderlen as early as 1911 (32). Some of these early attempts were based on the physiological studies of Weed as well as laboratory animal studies by innovative researchers including Harvey Cushing (19, 26).

While some surgeons were working with ventriculovenous bypass, others chose to explore pleural (Heile, 1914) (49) and lumbar (Ferguson, 1898) (34) or ventricular (Kausch, 1908) (57) to peritoneal diversion. Ferguson had little success with implementation of a silver wire passed between lumbar theca and peritoneum, and Kausch attributed the rapid demise of his patient to overdrainage via ventriculoperitoneal conduit. In 1898 Nicoll (83) suggested a paravertebral approach to the peritoneum, drawing up a free edge of omentum with attachment to a defect in the spinal dura.

Cushing (17) connected the subarachnoid space to the peritoneal or retroperitioneal spaces via simultaneous laparotomy and laminectomy, passing silver cannulae through holes in the L4 vertebral body. By 1908 12 patients were reported with "a considerable measure of success" (18). Some infants subsequently developed intussusception, which was erroneously attributed (26) to pituitary secretions in the CSF.

Heile (48) and others attempted to drain fluid into the peritoneal cavity by sewing the serosal surface of a loop of intestine to a slit in the spinal dura or introducing silk thread from the subarachnoid space to the peritoneum. Heile also tried saphenous vein and latex rubber conduits between the subarachnoid space and peritoneum (49). An 11-year-old boy was reported to have had such a tube inserted at the age of 5 months, and although the boy was living and well he had extruded the rubber tube practically every year (50). Heile should also be recognized for early attempts to divert the subarachnoid fluid to the urinary drainage system (50). About 1925 he accomplished this in four patients by anastomosis of the subarachnoid space to the renal pelvis after nephrectomy.

By 1929, Davidoff could report that the mechanics of the CSF and its pathological alterations were becoming better understood. He commented both on the improved understanding of the reaction of the body to newly established pathways and foreign materials, and on the eventual imperviousness of serosal surfaces to CSF. He speculated on the safety of allowing CSF to pour into the peritoneal cavity but added that a large number of cases had been "cured" by spinal-peritoneostomy. He reasoned that new types of autologous conduits would be have to be devised (26).

In 1963, Scarff (103) reviewed 20th century therapeutic advances in the treatment of hydrocephalus, and paid special tribute to Walter Dandy, who "almost single-handed, established the true pathology of hydrocephalus and developed sound physiological principles for its treatment." Dandy's contributions were truly impressive. With Blackfan he demonstrated that CSF is formed within the ventricles primarily by the choroid plexus (21). He refined our understanding of CSF circulation and described what modern clinicians would call noncommunicating and communicating hydrocephalus, devising the phenolsulfonphthein (PSP) intraventricular dye test to distinguish between them. The appearance of the phenolsulfonphthalein dye instilled into the ventricle in the lumbar CSF indicated free communication of these spaces and that no block existed within the ventricular system. This test was widely used by neurosurgeons to determine their approach to treatment (40). Until Dandy conceived and described ventriculography in 1918 (22), there was no certain method to confirm the diagnosis of hydrocephalus or to determine sites of CSF obstruction.

In 1919, Dandy introduced choroid plexectomy to attempt to reduce CSF formation (25). Open choroid plexectomy was hazardous because of the extensive collapse of the cerebral hemispheres, however, and Putnam (96) and Scarff (102) acted upon Dandy's suggestion to introduce endoscopic cauterization of the plexus. This method was widely applied before 1950. In 1963 Scarff (103) reviewed his own cases and those from the literature, concluding from 524 cases that operative mortality (15%) was similar to most other procedures of the day. Arrest of hydrocephalus was achieved in 71% but the procedure is no longer carried out because of the subsequent discovery of significant extra-choroidal sources of CSF (94).

Third ventriculostomy was introduced to bypass the obstruction to CSF flow due to aqueduct occlusion, but beginning with callosalsubarachnoidostomy in 1908 and Dandy's subfrontal and subtemporal approaches, mortality remained quite high. Subsequent endoscopic procedures, the through-and-through subfrontal method of Stookey and Scarff (112), and Dandy's later subtemporal and frontal approaches reduced third ventriculostomy mortality rates to 15%; 70% of patients surviving appeared to have arrest of their hydrocephalus.

Intracranial CSF diversion with newly directed artifical conduits seems to have been initiated by Torkildsen (113) before 1939. Small plastic or rubber tubes were led from the lateral ventricles extracranially and subcutaneously back to the cisterna magna. From subsequent accounts the success rate was nearly comparable to that of third ventriculostomy and plexus cauterization, but the operative mortality was initially twice as high (30%). Many other neurosurgeons have employed internal conduits to cisternal and similar subarachnoid sites (103), and a number of these procedures were used in the control of hydrocephalus associated with intracranial tumor. The Torkildsen shunt and its offspring have largely succumbed to the standard extracranial diversion procedures used today. Attempts to produce permanent internal fistulae by endoscopic or stereotactic methods have been revived in the 1970's and 1980's.

An extensive experience with ventricular and lumbar subarachnoid shunting to the ureter was reported from the Boston Children's Hospital by Matson in 1949 (69) and 1956 (70). Although operative mortality was nil, the procedure required a nephrectomy. Complications, both obstructive and infectious, and the predisposition of patients to dehydration and electrolyte imbalance, limited its application and dictated eventual abandonment of ureteral drainage. To the credit of Matson and his colleagues, a number of patients continue to survive 20 to 30 years after ureteral diversion.

Medical therapy for hydrocephalus continued to play a role throughout the 20th century (Table 1.1). Early in this century thyroid extract was thought to depress choroid plexus production of CSF. This substance (30, 40, 44) as well as the diuretic theobromine sodium salicylate (68), was used in many patients between 1906 and 1925. In spite of several encouraging reports of success, interest waned with the introduction of new surgical procedures.

This second era in the treatment of hydrocephalus owed much to the emergence of physiological studies, antiseptic and aseptic practices, and the development of neurological surgery as a specific discipline. Improved understanding of the pathology of hydrocephalus exemplified by the contributions of Dorothy Russell (100) should not go without recognition.

THE MODERN ERA: 1950-1989

This third and current epoch in the evolution of therapy has derived from advanced use of fabricated plastic substances with antireflux valves. Working with John Holter, a dedicated, skillful layman and father of a hydrocephalic child, Nulsen and Spitz (85) in Philadelphia implanted newly designed devices in the internal jugular vein and right cardiac atrium. Although the prototypes were constructed of polyvinyl chloride, silicone soon came to their attention as a potentially implantable, sterilizable substance. Almost simultaneously in California, Pudenz (93) produced an experimental one-way slit valve system molded of silicone. This was first tried in animals and rapidly taken to the clinic where it was inserted in a patient as a ventriculoatrial (VA) shunt in 1955. Ingraham and his associates (55) conceived the usefulness of polyethylene and with laboratory experiments had seemingly proven its potential as an implant in biological systems. Matson's meticulous approaches with ureteral shunts paralleled these other efforts (71). Cone, who never published on the subject, has been widely recognized for the introduction of peritoneal shunts using plastics during part of this period (95, 116). Ransohoff treated a number of patients with subdural to pleural diversion using red rubber catheters (99).

These efforts, especially the techniques of Nulsen and Spitz and Pudenz, heralded the rapid development of commercially manufactured shunts, which generated the relatively standardized practices of today. Peritoneal diversion was again attempted (56, 81) with in-

TABLE 1.2.
Biological and Foreign Materials and Receptacle Sites in CSF Diversion.

Material	Device
Glass wool	'nail'
Gold	Tube
Silver	Tube, coiled wire
Platinum	Tube
Glass	Tube
Linen	Strand
Catgut	Strand
Silk	Strand
Cargile membrane	Strand
Rubber	Tube
Latex	Tube
Vein graft	Tube
Calves arteries	Tube
'Plastic'	Tube, strip
Omentum	Strip
Portex	Tube
Tigon	Tube
Polyethylene	Tube, valve
Polyvinyl chloride	Tube, valve
Silicone	Tube, valve

Extracranial Receptacle Sites	Intracranial Receptacle Sites
Subgaleal	Subdural
Subcutaneous-face	Subarachnoid
Mastoid	Interventricular
Salivary ducts	
Peritoneal	*Intraspinal*
Retroperitoneal	Extradural
Orbit	Bone marrow
Kidney	
Ureter	*Vascular*
Pleural	Sagittal sinus
Thoracic duct	Torcular
Retromental	Jugular vein
Stomach	Superficial temporal vein
Gallbladder	Cardiac atrium
Ileum	(indirect, direct)
Fallopian tube	

thoracic (lymphatic) duct (120), fallopian tube (46), gallbladder (108), spinal epidural space (45), salivary ducts (89), stomach (2, 64) and ileum (82) (Table 1.2). Long-term results of the majority of these procedures, as for direct heart shunting (86), have rarely been published.

Ventriculoperitoneal (VP) shunting was resurrected by Ames (4) and by Raimondi and Matsumoto (98), using improved silicone devices. The revitalization of VP shunting was welcomed by many surgeons struggling with the requirement for frequent lengthening of the atrial shunts (8, 37, 60) in growing children. During the past two decades an enormous array of hardware has been developed for the relatively simple task of VP diversion. Some devices have been ingenious, and others cumbersome and trouble-prone. The compendium includes various size proximal and distal slit valves; proximal diaphragm and spring-ball valves; numerous reservoirs, antisiphon devices, and antechambers; plain, flanged, curved, and slotted ventricular catheters; spring-reinforced tubes; kink-resistant silicone tubes; expandable systems to accommodate axial growth; and implantable telemetric pressure sensors (73, 92). Lumboperitoneal shunting has been repopularized with the adding of percutaneous technique, small-bore silicone tubes, and ingenious valve systems (111).

During the 1950's and 1960's conscientious, dedicated investigators were able to develop this technology in a relatively unencumbered medical environment, but contemporary innovation is not nearly so easy. The introduction of new designs has come under extensive government scrutiny. Recently a standard governing the design and production of shunt equipment has been promulgated (3).

Coincident with evolution of CSF shunts, surgeons have continued to describe technological applications aimed at curing, rather than simply controlling the condition. Direct attacks on the cerebral aqueduct (23, 25, 66) are periodically reported, but surgical mortality and morbidity remain high. Elvidge, reporting in 1966, took up Dandy's aqueduct cannulation procedure on 10 older patients in whom he recorded a 20% operative mortality (31). Considerable clinical improvement was noted in survivors, although early pneumoencephalograms seemed to show persistent severe ventriculomegaly.

different results, and polyethylene tubing was eventually found to be inadequate for the task. Pleural shunting declined because of chronic pleural effusion and shunt obstruction. Lumboperitoneal shunting via laminectomy using polyethylene tubes fell into disrepute because of the risk of scoliosis (63). VA shunting became a standard practice (94) in the 1960's, a time when various innovative surgeons described small series of procedures using diverse CSF absorption sites including the subdural space (36), mastoid process (84),

Reporting in the same issue of the Journal of Neurosurgery, fellow Canadians Turnbull and Drake documented impressive results with perforations of membranous veils of the aqueduct in 4 children (114). Intervention was supported by careful preoperative radiographic contrast studies. This type of anatomical definition may again become possible in our current noninvasive diagnostic climate with the proliferation of MRI.

Crosby and his colleagues were among the last to recommend direct cannulation of the aqueduct (16). In 1973 they described a series of 30 infants in whom flared silastic tubes were placed in the aqueduct after preoperative decompression with ventriculoatrial shunts. Two expired with early CSF fistulae and meningitis. Seven others died 1 month to 3 years later. Among survivors 63% were judged to have surgical arrest of the condition.

Improved endoscopic and stereotaxic procedures continue to find application in hydrocephalus. The most recent return to aqueductal cannulation by Backlund and colleagues (7) employed stereotaxy. Seven patients had 13 stereotaxic procedures for positioning of an aqueductal prosthesis, with control of hydrocephalus in 4 patients.

Third ventriculostomy, although certainly not competitive with extracranial diversionary methods, has experienced a revival with refined technology. Sayers and Kosnik (101) and Hoffman and associates (54) have each contributed to the preparation and rationale for selection of candidates, advocating preoperative extracranial CSF diversion and assessment of potential extraventricular CSF pathways. Vries (115) has revived the method of Mixter (78), using a precise endoscopic system for third ventriculostomy, but continuing problems with patient selection plague this technique. The ease and standardization of certain conventional procedures such as VP shunting tend to inhibit the introduction and testing of these newer and less predictable treatments.

Medical therapies for hydrocephalus resurface periodically. Since 1950 limited series of cases have been treated with a number of diuretics, including the osmotic agents sucrose, glycerol, isosorbide, and urea (118). The carbonic anhydrase inhibiter acetazolamide has been used alone or in combination with furosemide for temporary and in some cases for long-term control of hydrocephalus. The most recent experience involves temporization with medical measures for preterm neonates who may eventually achieve compensation of posthemorrhagic hydrocephalus (106).

Selection of patients, guidance for management, and monitoring of the hydrocephalic condition have been remarkably facilitated by the imaging techniques introduced during the past 15 years. Wide application of CT, cranial sonography (for infants with open fontanelles), and the newer MRI has undeniably revolutionized diagnosis, selection for treatment, and evaluation of progress in hydrocephalic patients (73). Radionuclide, air, and postive-contrast media procedures are now infrequently used or required.

The results of early therapy of hydrocephalus with valve-regulated silicone systems were distressingly similar to the recorded natural history of the condition. Complications were numerous and occasionally fatal. However, the neurosurgical record has gradually reflected what has become an impressive reversal in the mortality as well as the functional capacity of survivors with shunt-treated hydrocephalus (60). Laurence and Coates (65) documented a 46% 10-year survival rate and intellectual disability in 62% of untreated children in 1962. Mealey et al. reported a similar result after short-term follow-up in congential hydrocephalics treated with VA shunts (74). Foltz and Shurtleff (35) provided one of the first encouraging reports of treated patients in 1963. Subsequently, the 10-year survival rate has approached 95% and intellectual deficit afflicts about 30% of pediatric patients (76). However, complex functional deficits are common even among survivors with normal intelligence (29). Shunt revision rates in this population approximate 2 per patient for the first 10 years after insertion. For adult hydrocephalus there are continuing problems with patient selection as well as morbidity (72). Indications for therapy of the "normal" pressure (1) variety of hydrocephalus remain controversial, but for acute adult types and those with noncommunicating hydrocephalus and increased intracranial pressure, there has been undoubted benefit.

In the present era, hydrocephalus is fairly reliably controlled but cures remain few and far between. Given its multiple etiologies, it seems likely that the treatment of hydrocephalus will remain a problem for future neurosurgeons. Therefore the rationale for continuing improvement of CSF diversionary systems is well-founded; prevention of overdrainage and maintenance of optimum intracranial pressure in the shunted child are only a few of the problems to be solved (72). Although infection rates are declining, consistently reliable measures to prevent shunt infection must be sought. Improved operative techniques and materials will undoubtedly decrease the number of shunt revisions required because of growth or device breakage.

REFERENCES

1. Adams, R.D., Fisher, C.M., Hakim, S., *et al.* Symptomatic occult hydrocephalus with "normal" cerebrospinal fluid pressure. A treatable syndrome. New. Engl. J. Med. *273:*117–126, 1965.
2. Alther, E. Dasmagenventil. Eineneue operation methode zur behandlung des kindlichen hydrocephalus. Schweiz. Med. Wochenschr. 95:234–236, 1965.
3. American Society for Testing Materials Standards F 647-79: Standard practice for evaluating and specifying implantable shunting assemblies for neurosurgical application, Philadelphia, 1980.
4. Ames, R.H. Ventriculoperitoneal shunts in the management of hydrocephalus. J. Neurosurg. 27:525–529, 1967.
5. Andrews, E.W. An improved technique in brain surgery; glass tubes versus gold or platinum for subdural drainage of the lateral ventricles in internal hydrocephalus. Trans. Am. Surg. Assoc. 29:111–1911.
6. Anton, G., von Bramann, F. Balkenstich bei hydrozephalien, tumoren und bei epilepsie. Munchen med. Wchnschr. 55:1673–1677, 1908.
7. Backlund, E.O., Grepe, A., and Lunsford, D. Stereotaxic reconstruction of the aqueduct of Sylvius. J. Neurosurg. 55:800–810, 1981.
8. Becker, D.P. and Nulsen, F.E. Control of hydrocephalus by valve-regulated venous shunt: avoidance of complications in prolonged shunt maintenance. J. Neurosurg. 28:215–226, 1968.
9. Bennett, J.R. *The Causes Nature, Diagnosis and Treatment of Acute Hydrocephalus or Water in the Head.* p. 248, London, Samuel Highley, 1843.
10. Bering, E. A. Jr. Problems of the dynamics of the cerebrospinal fluid with particular reference to the formation of cerebrospinal fluid and its relationship to cerebral metabolism. Clin. Neurosurg. 5:77–97, 1958.
11. Boerhaave. *Aphorism,* 1218 (cited by Whytt, p. 5) (119).
12. Brainard. 1825 (cited by Davidoff, p. 1739) (26).
13. von Bramann, F. Die behandlung des hydrocephalus durch Balkenstich. Deutsche med. Wchnschr. 35:1645–1647, 1909.
14. Broca, A. Drainage des ventricules cerebraux pour hydrocephalic. Rev. Chir. *11:*37–52, 1891.
15. Cotungo, D. *De Ischiade Nervosa Commentaries.* Naples, Fratus Simonios, 1764.
16. Crosby, R.M.N., Henderson, C.M., and Paul, R.L. Catheterization of the cerebral aqueduct for obstructive hydrocephalus in infants. J. Neurosurg. *38:*596–601, 1973.
17. Cushing, H. The special field of neurological surgery. Cleveland Med. J. *4:*1–25, 1905.
18. Cushing, H. The Cerebral Envelopes. In: *SURGERY*, Vol. 3, edited by W. W. Keen, p. 111, Philadelphia, W.B. Saunders, 1908.
19. Cushing, H. *Studies in Intracranial Physiology and Surgery* (lecture I, third circulation). London, Humphrey Milford, 1926.
20. Cutler, R.W.P., Page, L., and Galicich, J. Formation and absorption of cerebrospinal fluid in man. Brain *91:*707–720, 1968.
21. Dandy, W.E., and Blackfan, K.D. Internal hydrocephalus. An experimental, clinical and pathological study. Am J. Dis. Child 8:406–482, 1914.
22. Dandy, W.E. Ventriculostomy following the injection of air into the cerebral ventricles. Ann. Surg. 68:5–11, 1918.
23. Dandy, W.E. The diagnosis and treatment of hydrocephalus resulting from strictures of the aqueduct of Sylvius. Surg. Gynecol. Obst. *31:*340–358, 1920.
24. Dandy, W.E. The diagnosis and treatment of hydrocephalus due to occlusions of the foramina of Magendie and Luschka. Surg. Gynecol. Obst. *32:*112–124, 1921.
25. Dandy, W.E. Diagnosis and Treatment of Strictures of the aqueduct of Sylvius (causing hydrocephalus). Arch. Surg. *51:*1–14, 1945.
26. Davidoff, L.M. Treatment of hydrocephalus. Historical review and description of a new method. Arch. Surg. *18:*1737–1762, 1929.
27. Davson, H. *Physiology of the Cerebrospinal Fluid.* London, Churchill, 1967.
28. Denk, W. Zur chirurgie des liquer-systems. Wien. Klin. Wochenschr. 40:1349–1357, 1927.
29. Dennis, M., Fitz, C.R., Netley C.T., *et al.* The intelligence of hydrocephalic children. Arch. Neurol. *38:*607–615, 1981.
30. Elsberg, C.A. Chronic internal hydrocephalus: the newer methods for its recognition and treatment. Med. Rec. 92:874–875, 1917.
31. Elvidge, A.R. Treatment of obstructive lesions of the aqueduct of Sylvius and the fourth ventricle by interventriculostomy. J. Neurosurg. 24:11–23, 1966.
32. Enderlen, E. Zur behandlung des hydrocephalus. Beitr. Klin. Chir. 76:889–890, 1911.
33. Epstein, F., Wald, A., and Hochwald, G.M. Intracranial pressure during compressive head wrapping in treatment of neonatal hydrocephalus. Pediatrics 54:786–790, 1974.
34. Ferguson, A.H. (Editorial) New York Med. J. 1:902, 1898. Cited by Davidoff (26), p. 1748.
35. Foltz, E.L., and Shurtleff, D.B. Five year comparative study of hydrocephalus in children with and without operation (113 cases). J. Neurosurg. 20:1065–1078, 1963.
36. Forrest, D.M., Laurence, K.M., and Mcnab, G.H. Ventriculosubdura! drainage in infantile hydrocephalus. Analysis of early results. Lancet 2:1274–1277, 1957.
37. Forrest, D.M., and Cooper, D.G.W. Complications of ventriculo-atrial shunts. A review of 455 cases. J. Neurosurg 29:506–512, 1968.

38. Fowler, R.S. The surgical treatment of internal hydrocephalus. Ann. Surg. 49:374–381, 1909.
39. Fraser, J., and Dott, N.M. Hydrocephalus Br. J. Surg. 10:165–191, 1922–23.
40. Frazier, C.H. Types of hydrocephalus—their differentiation and treatment. Am. J. Dis. Child 11:95–102, 1916.
41. Fuller, C.K. Some observations on chronic hydrocephalus with report of a case apparently arrested. Can. Med. Assoc. J, 17:675–677, 1927.
42. Glynn, Thomas J. Case of hydrocephalus; trephining; opening of fourth ventricle; recovery. Lancet 2:1106, 1895.
43. Goldstein, G., Chaplin, E., and Maitland, J. Transient hydrocephalus in premature infants: treatment by lumbar punctures. Lancet 1:512–514, 1976.
44. Gray, J.P. Administration of thyroid gland in hydrocephalus. Lancet 2:177, 1922.
45. Hakim, S., Jimenez, Z., and Rosas, F. Drainage of cerebrospinal fluid into the spinal epidural space. Acta Neurochir. 4:224–227, 1955.
46. Harsh, G.H. Peritoneal shunt for hydrocephalus. Utilizing the fimbria of the fallopian tube for entrance to the peritoneal cavity. J. Neurosurg. 11:284–294, 1954.
47. Haynes, I.S. Congentital internal hydrocephalus. Its treatment by drainage of the cisterna magna into cranial sinuses. Ann. Surg. 57:449–484, 1913.
48. Heile, B. Zur behandling des hydrocephalus. Deutsche med. Wchnschr. 24:1468–1470, 1908.
49. Heile, B. Zur chirugischen behandlung des hydrocephalus internus durch ableitting der cerebrospinal flussikeit nach der bauchhole und nach der pleurakuppe. Arch. Klin. Chir. 105:501–516, 1914.
50. Heile, B. Ueber neue operative wege zur drucken Hastung bei angeborenen hydrocephalus (ureter-duraanastomose). Zentralbl. Chir. 52:2229–2236, 1925.
51. Hieronymus Mercurialis, Cited by Whytt (119), p. 5.
52. Hildenbrand, O. Eine-neue operations-method zur behandlung des hydrocephalus internus chronicus der kinder. Arch Klin. Chir. 127:178–194, 1923.
53. Hippocrates. De Morbis. Cited by Whytt (119), p. 4.
54. Hoffman, H.J., Harwood-Nash, D., and Gilday, D.L. Percutaneous third ventriculostomy in the management of noncommunicating hydrocephalus. Neurosurgery 7:313–321, 1980.
55. Ingraham, F.D., Alexander, E. Jr., and Matson, D.D. Synthetic plastic material in surgery. N. Eng. J. Med. 236:362–367, 402–407, 1947.
56. Jackson, I.J., and Snodgrass, S.R. Peritoneal shunts in the treatment of hydrocephalus and increased intracranial pressure. J. Neurosurg. 12:216–222, 1955.
57. Kausch, W. Die behandlung des hydrocephalus der Kleinen Kinder. Arch. Klin. Chir. 87:709–796, 1908.
58. Keen, W.W. Surgery of the lateral ventricles. Verhandl d X internat med Kongr iii, Chirurgie, Berlin, p. 108, 1891.
59. Kempe, L.G., and Blaylock, R. Ventriculolymphatic shunt. J. Neurosurg. 47:86–95, 1977.
60. Keucher, T.R., and Mealey, J. Jr. Long-term results after ventriculoatrial and ventriculoperitoneal shunt for infantile hydrocephalus. J. Neurosurg. 50:179–186, 1979.
61. Key, E.A.H., and Retzius, G. Studien in der Anatomie des Nervensystems and des Bindegewebes. Stockholm, Samson & Wallin, 1875.
62. Krause, F. Subcutane dauerdrainage der hirnventrikel beim hydrocephalus. Verhendl d. Berlin med. Gesellsch. 39:213, 1908–1909.
63. Kushner, J., Alexander, E. Jr., and Davis, C.H. Kyphoscoliosis following lumbar subarachnoid shunts. J. Neurosurg. 34:783–791, 1971.
64. Lamesch, A.J. Ventriculogastrostomy by means of a gastric tube for the treatment of hydrocephalus. A preliminary report. J. Pediatr. Surg. 7:55–59, 1972.
65. Laurence, K.M., and Coates, S. The natural history of hydrocephalus. Detailed analysis of 182 unoperated cases. Arch. Dis. Child 37:345–362, 1962.
66. Leksell, L. A surgical procedure for atresia of the aqueduct of Sylvius. Acta Psychiat. Neurol. Scand. 24:559–568, 1949.
67. Magendie, F. Memoire sur le liquide qui se trouve dans le crane et l'e'pine del'homme and des animaux. J. Physiol. Exp. Path. 5:27–37, 1825.
68. Marriott, W.M. The use of theobromin sodiosalicylate (diuretic) in treatment of hydrocephalus. Am. J. Dis. Child 28:479–483, 1924.
69. Matson, D.D. New operation for treatment of communicating hydrocephalus: report of case secondary to generalized meningitis. J. Neurosurg. 6:238–247, 1949.
70. Matson, D.D. Current treatment of hydrocephalus. New. Engl. J. Med. 255:933–936, 1956.
71. Matson, D.D. The surgical treatment of hydrocephalus. In: Disorders of the Developing Nervous System, edited by W.S. Fields, pp 483–488, Springfield IL, Thomas, 1961.
72. McCullough, D.C., and Fox, J.L. Negative intracranial pressure hydrocephalus in adults with shunts and its relationship to the production of subdural hematoma. J. Neurosurg. 40:372–375, 1974.
73. McCullough, D.C. A history of the treatment of hydrocephalus. Fetal Therapy 1:38–45, 1986.
74. Mealey, J. Jr., Gilmore, R.L., and Bubb, M.P. The prognosis of hydrocephalus overt at birth. J. Neurosurg. 39:348–355, 1973.
75. Miculicz J. Cited by Davidoff (26), p. 1741.
76. Milhorat, T.H. Hydrocephalus and the Cerebrospinal Fluid. Baltimore, Williams & Wilkins, p. 178, 1972.
77. Milhorat, T.H. Hydrocephalus: historical notes, etiology and clinical diagnosis. In: Pediatric Neurosurgery, edited by R.L. McLauren, pp. 197–210, New York, Grune & Stratton, 1984.
78. Mixter, W.J. Ventriculostomy and puncture of the third ventricle. Boston Med. Surg. J. 188:277–278, 1923.
79. Morgagne, G.B. The Seats and Causes of Diseases Investigated by Anatomy, London, Miller & Cadell, 1761.
80. Murphey, Cited by Davidoff (26), p 1745.
81. Murtagh, F., and Lehman, R. Peritoneal shunts in the management of hydrocephalus. J.A.M.A. 202:1010–1014, 1967.

82. Neumann, C.G., Hoen, T.I., and Davis, D.A. The adaption of ileoentectropy to the control of communicating hydrocephalus. Plast Reconstr. Surg. 23:159–167, 1959.

83. Nicoll, J.H. Case of hydrocephalus in which peritoneo-meningeal drainage has been carried out. Glasgow Med. J. 63:187–191, 1905.

84. Nosik, W.A. Ventriculomastoidostomy. Technique and observations. J. Neurosurg. 7:236–239, 1950.

85. Nulsen, F.E., and Spitz, E.B. Treatment of hydrocephalus by direct shunt from ventricle to jugular vein. Surg. Forum 2:399–403, 1952.

86. Overton, M.C. III, Snodgrass, S.R., and Derrick, J.R. Direct atrial and vena caval shunting procedures for hydrocephalus. Surg. Gynecol. Obstet. 124:819–825, 1965.

87. Pappenheimer, J.R., Heisey, S.R., and Jordan, E.F. Perfusion of the ventricular system in unanesthetized goats. Am. J. Physiol. 203:763–774, 1962.

88. Parkin, A. The treatment of chronic hydrocephalus by basal drainage. Lancet 2:1244, 1893.

89. Parkinson, D., and Jain, K.K. Hydrocephalus. A shunt between the ventricle and Stensen's duct. Can. J. Surg. 4:183–185, 1961.

90. Payr, E. Drainage der Hirnventrikel mittelst frei transplantirter Blutgefasse; Bemerkungen ueber Hydrocephalus. Arch. Klin. Chir. 87:801–885, 1908.

91. Payr, E. Ueber Ventrikeldrainage bei Hydrocephalus. Verh dt Ges Chir 40:515–535, 1911.

92. Portnoy, H.D. Hydrodynamics of shunts. In. Monographs in Neural Sciences, edited by M.M. Cohen, Vol. 8, Basel, Karger, pp. 179–183, 1982.

93. Pudenz, R.H., Russell, F.E., and Hurd, A.H., et al. Ventriculoauriculostomy. A technique for shunting cerebrospinal fluid into the right auricle. Preliminary report. J. Neurosurg. 14:171–179, 1957.

94. Pudenz, R.H. The surgical treatment of hydrocephalus. In Disorders of the Developing Nervous System, edited by W.S. Fields, pp. 468–489, Springfield IL, Thomas, 1961.

95. Pudenz, R.H. The surgical treatment of hydrocephalus—an historical review. Surg. Neurol. 15:15–26, 1980.

96. Putnam, T. The surgical treatment of infantile hydrocephalus. Surg. Gynecol. Obstet 76:171–182, 1943.

97. Quincke, H. Ueber Hydrocephalus. Verh. Congr. inn. Med. 10:321–339, 1891.

98. Raimondi, A.J., and Matsumoto, S. A simplified technique for performing the ventriculoperitoneal shunt. (Technical note). J. Neurosurg. 26:357–360, 1967.

99. Ransohoff, J. Ventriculopleural anastomosis in treatment of midline obstructional neoplasms. J. Neurosurg. 11:295–298, 1954.

100. Russell, D.S. Observations on the Pathology of Hydrocephalus. (Special Report Series Number 265, Medical Research Council) London, Her Majesty's Stationary Office, 1949.

101. Sayers, M.P., and Kosnik, E.J. Percutaneous third ventriculostomy: experience and technique. Child's Brain 2:24–30, 1976.

102. Scarff, J.E. Nonobstructive hydrocephalus. Treatment by endoscopic cauterization of the choroid plexuses. Am. J. Dis. Child 63:297–334, 1942.

103. Scarff, J.E. Treatment of hydrocephalus: an historical and critical review of methods and results. J. Neurol. Neurosurg. Psychiatry 26:1–26, 1963.

104. Sgalitzer, M. Neue Erkenntnisse auf dem Gebieteder Rontgenstrahlenwirkung bei Hirntumoren. Strahlentherapie 22:701–708, 1926.

105. Sharpe, W. The operative treatment of hydrocephalus; A preliminary report on forty-one patients. Am. J. Med. Sci. 153:563–571,1917.

106. Shinnar, S., Gammon, K., Bergman, E.W., et al. Management of hydrocephalus in infancy: Use of acetazolamide and furosemide to avoid cerebrospinal fluid shunts. J. Pediatr. 107:31–37, 1985.

107. Siedamgrotsky. Beeinthissung der Production des Ventrikelliquor durch Roentgenbestrahlung der Plexus choroidei. Arch & Klin. Chir. 145:122–127, 1927.

108. Smith, G.W., Moretz, W.H., and Pritchard, W.L. Ventriculobiliary shunt. A new treatment for hydrocephalus. Surg. Forum 9:701–705, 1959.

109. Sokolowski, M., and Irger, J. Dielympangioplastik des unterhorns des seiter ventikels des behandlungs method beihydrocephalus internus. Zentralblf. Chir. 52:2586–2589, 1925.

110. Somma. Cited by Davidoff (26), p. 1739.

111. Spetzler, R., Wilson, C.B., and Schulte R. Simplified percutaneous lumboperitoneal shunting. Surg. Neurol. 7:25–29, 1977.

112. Stookey, B., and Scarff, J. Occlusion of the aqueduct of Sylvius by neoplastic and non-neoplastic processes with a rational surgical treatment for relief of the resultant obstructive hydrocephalus. Bull. Neurol. Inst. N.Y. 5:348–377, 1936.

113. Torkildsen, A. A new palliative operation in cases of inoperable occlusion of the sylvian aqueduct. Acta Chir. Scand. 82:117–125, 1939.

114. Turnbull, I.M., and Drake, C.G. Membranous occlusion of the aqueduct of Sylvius. J. Neurosurg. 24:24–33, 1966.

115. Vries, J. An endoscopic technique for third ventriculostomy. Surg. Neurol. 9:165–168, 1978.

116. Wallman, L.J. Shunting for hydrocephalus: an oral history. Neurosurgery 11:308–313, 1982.

117. Weed, L.H. Certain anatomical and physiological aspects of the meninges and cerebrospinal fluid. Brain 58:383–397, 1935.

118. Welch, K. The principles of physiology of the cerebrospinal fluid in relation to hydrocephalus including normal pressure hydrocephalus. In: Advances in Neurology, Vol. 13, edited by W.J. Freelander, pp. 247–332, New York, Raven Press, 1975.

119. Whytt, R. Observations on the Dropsy in the Brain. Edinburgh, J. Balfour, 1768.

120. Yokoyama, I., Aoki, H., Takebayashi, K., et al. Ventriculolymphangiostomy. A shunting operation for hydrocephalus to drain cerebrospinal fluid into the thoracic duct. Folia Psychiatr. Neurol. Jpn. 13:305–319, 1959.

CHAPTER 2

Current Concepts of CSF Production and Absorption

HAROLD REKATE, M.D., and
WILLIAM OLIVERO, M.D.

INTRODUCTION

Cerebrospinal fluid (CSF) production and absorption are in a dynamic equilibrium, with average production equaling average absorption under normal physiological conditions. Intrinsic compensatory mechanisms allow for changes in production and absorption to be tolerated; however, when these mechanisms are blocked or overwhelmed, pathological conditions involving the CSF occur. The anatomy and physiology of these processes will be examined.

ANATOMY

Most CSF (50%-80%) is produced by the choroid plexus that lines the walls of the lateral ventricles and roof of the third and fourth ventricles (43, 40, 62, 4). The importance of various extrachoroidal sources of CSF is unclear (45). Plexectomized animals continue to secrete CSF, and hydrocephalus develops in these animals if the foramen of Monro or aqueduct of Sylvius is blocked (41). Plexectomy as a treatment for hydrocephalus in humans is uniformly unsuccessful except as a temporizing measure (44, 45, 13), and Milhorat et al (46) have reported a normal rate of CSF production in a patient 5 years postplexectomy. However, plexectomy involves only the lateral ventricles, leaving the choroid plexus in the third and fourth ventricles as sources of CSF. When Pollay et al (53) perfused the ependyma of the rabbit from the aqueduct of Sylvius to the anterior fourth ventricle (thereby excluding the choroid plexus), their results suggested that as much as 30% of the CSF may come from the brain's ependymal surface. However, their experimental design

required extensive surgical manipulation that may have influenced the results.

The brain parenchyma has been proposed as another possible source of CSF (43). Intracerebral injection studies suggest bulk flow of brain interstitial fluid in white matter (60). Cserr et al (9) have shown that compounds with different molecular weights were cleared from the brain relatively independent of their diffusion constants, suggesting bulk flow of fluid from the brain. Although early studies implicated the spinal subarachnoid space as a source of extrachoroidal CSF, more recent perfusion studies show little or no CSF production from this site (33, 61).

The choroid plexus is composed of villi, each with a connective tissue core covered by a single layer of cuboidal epithelium. Tight junctions are present on the apical surface of the epithelium with the basal surface having numerous infoldings (17, 18). These apical tight junctions are thought to represent the anatomical substrate of the blood-CSF barrier (Fig. 2.1) (6).

Choroidal CSF is formed as an ultrafiltrate from the capillaries in the center of each villus; this ultrafiltrate is processed by the choroidal epithelium, and secreted by diffusion into the ventricles. That choroidal CSF is secreted is supported by the differences found in the ionic composition of CSF compared to an ultrafiltrate of plasma (8). Pollay (54) has hypothesized the standing gradient to explain this secretory process. In this model, the ultrafiltrate from plasma enters the basal infoldings of the choroidal cells; Na^+ is then actively transported into the choroidal cells establishing an osmotic gradient and allowing free flow of water into the cell. A similar mechanism would

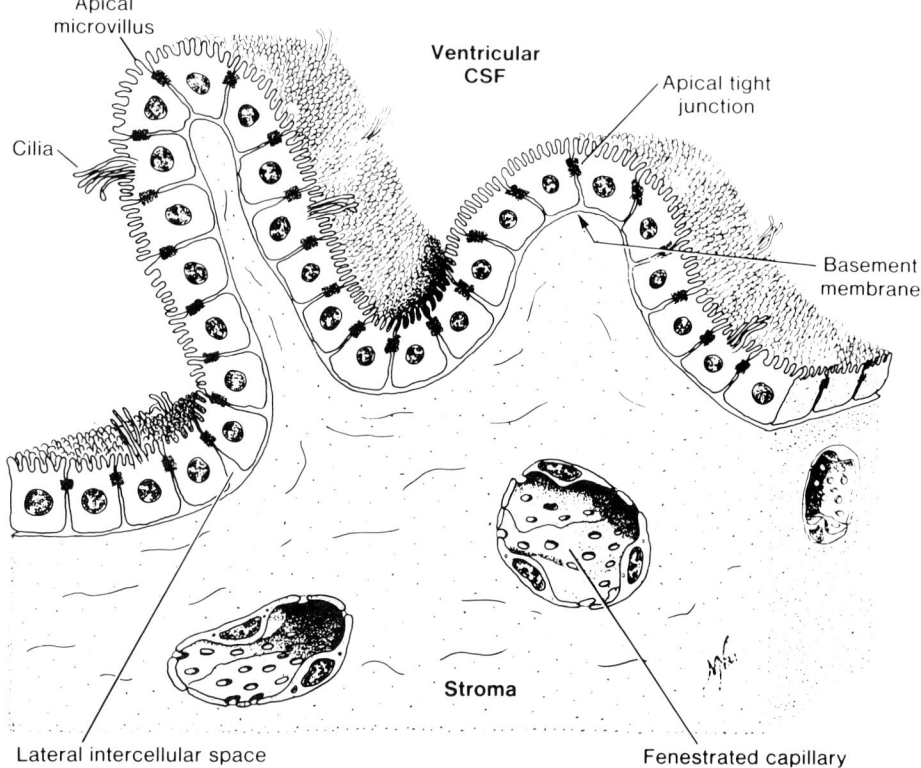

Figure 2.1. The anatomy of the choroidal epithelium demonstrating the apical tight junctions. (Reprinted with permission from M.B. Carpenter and J. Sutin, editors, *Human Neuroanatomy,* p. 22, Baltimore, Williams & Wilkins, 1983.)

then couple Na$^+$ and water movement into the ventricular system from the apical surface of the cell. An ATPase Na$^+$/K$^+$ pump is important in the secretory process and can be at least partially blocked by ouabain (55). Ouabain, a short-acting cardiac glycoside, is known to bind to the Na$^+$/K$^+$ ATPase and to block its function of Na$^+$/K$^+$ exchange. Acetazolamide, a carbonic anhydrase inhibitor, is known to decrease CSF production (73), but the exact role that the enzyme carbonic anhydrase plays in CSF secretion is unclear (54). Once formed, the CSF circulates throughout the ventricular system, exits the foramina of Magendie and Luschka in the fourth ventricle, circulates through the subarachnoid space of the spinal cord and brain, and is absorbed (Fig. 2.2).

The arachnoid villi have long been considered the primary site of CSF absorption (40, 45, 72). These are arachnoid diverticula that project into the veins and venous sinuses of the brain, the majority found along the superior sagittal sinus. Arachnoid granulations are villi visible to the unaided eye (70). Opinions are divided on exactly how CSF passes across these structures into the blood (15). One model envisions the existence of open channels through the arachnoid villi, functioning as one-way valves that allow passage of CSF but not retrograde flow of blood (15, 72). In the other model, there are no channels, the villi are covered by a continuous endothelial membrane, and passage of macromolecules would require an active transport process (2). Proponents of the open-channel model contend that the energy requirements would be too high for an active transport process to exist; however, several ultrastructural studies of the arachnoid villi have failed to reveal any channels (2, 64).

Recently, alternative sites of CSF absorption have received increased interest. McComb et al (39) found no arachnoid villi along the course of the rabbit's superior sagittal sinus, suggesting other routes for absorption. In obstructive hydrocephalus, where access to the arachnoid villi is largely blocked, the daily volumetric increase in ventricle size is much less than CSF production, suggesting alternative routes

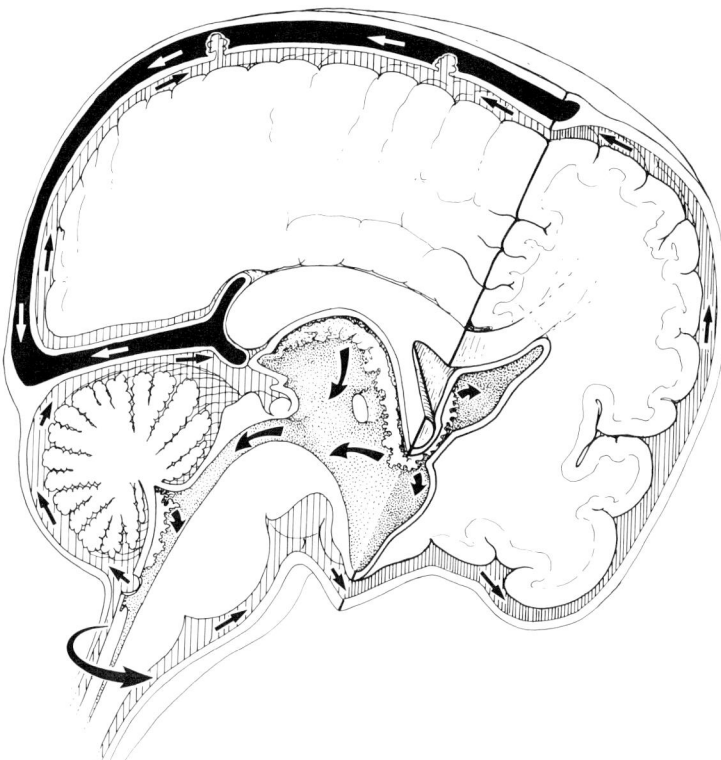

Figure 2.2.   The anatomy of the CSF pathways.

for absorption. Although the brain contains no true lymphatic channels, there is increasing evidence that lymphatic-type drainage of CSF does occur. By ligating cervical lymphatics in animals, Casley-Smith et al (7) have produced brain edema and dilatation of what they term the ''prelymphatic space'' around the cerebral blood vessels. They also observed that carbon injected into the brain can be traced into the cervical lymphatics. Other authors have documented passage of tracers along several of the cranial nerves, especially the olfactory, into the cervical lymph nodes (28). Foldi et al. (23) have noted that the blood-brain barrier is not absolute, and protein could accumulate within the brain unless lymphatics were available to eliminate it. Although lymphatic drainage of the brain has not been documented in humans, the increasing experimental evidence supporting the role of lymphatic drainage in other animals makes it a prime alternate or accessory site for CSF absorption in humans.

Brain capillaries are another possible site of CSF absorption. The periventricular hypodens-ity seen readily on computed tomography (CT) in the presence of active hydrocephalus has been assumed to indicate transependymal CSF absorption. That CSF enters the brain from the ventricle in hydrocephalus is well documented (26); however, this may not be equivalent to bulk flow of CSF into the brain capillaries. Eisenberg et al. (19) have argued that for bulk flow to occur, the pressure of the extracapillary CSF would have to be greater than the capillaries intraluminal pressure, thereby collapsing them. In fact, the brain may not function as an absorptive site for CSF but as a conduit to other sites (7, 19).

Paradoxically, the choroid plexus is another proposed site of CSF absorption. Milhorat (42) injected radioiodinated serum albumin into the lateral ventricles of 8 hydrocephalic children and measured the rate of change of the isotope from the ventricle before and after bilateral plexectomy. He found appreciable concentration of the tracer present in the removed choroid plexus, and after plexectomy, the rate of change of intraventricular isotope was re-

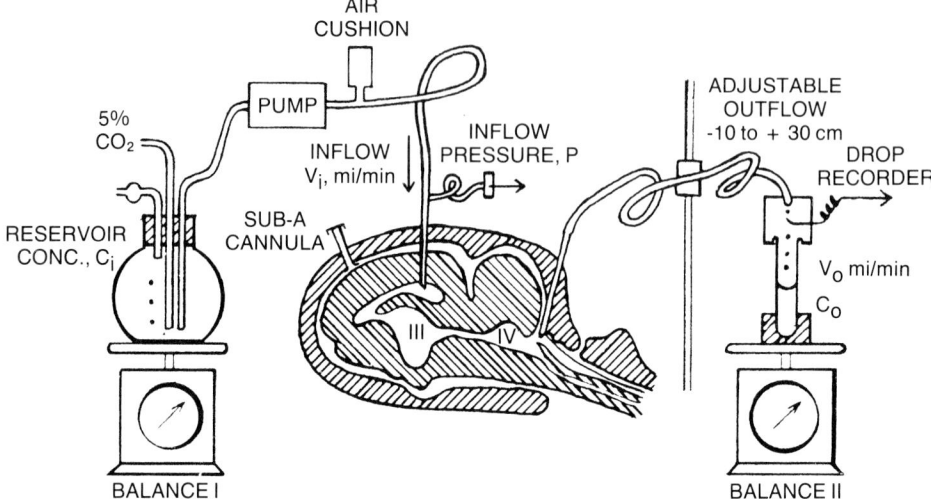

Figure 2.3. Diagram of perfusion system. Typical values for goats: brain wt. = 110 g; choroid plexuses = 500 mg; total CSF vol. = 25 ml; ventriculocisternal system = 10 ml; perfusion rate, V = 1-3 ml/min; rate of bulk formation of CSF = 0.15 ml/min. (Reprinted with permission from J.R. Pappenheimer, S.R. Heisey, E.F. Jordan, et al., *Perfusion of the Cerebral Ventricular System in Unanesthetized Goats.* Am. J. Physiol. 203(5):763–774, 1962.)

duced—both suggesting an absorptive role of the choroid plexus in hydrocephalus. Other experiments in Kaolin-induced hydrocephalus in cats yield conflicting results. These experiments failed to show any evidence of ventricular absorption during ventricular perfusion.

Dandy (11) postulated that most CSF absorption occurred diffusely from the subarachnoid space. At present, there does not appear to be significant evidence supporting this theory since under normal physiological conditions the arachnoid functions as a barrier to the egress of CSF.

It appears that the main site of CSF production is the choroid plexus, and that of absorption, the arachnoid villi; however, alternative sites exist for each process. How important they are in normal or disease states remains controversial.

PHYSIOLOGY

The flow of CSF depends on many interrelated phenomena. These include the rate of production, choroidal pulsations, resistance of the pathways, and absorption and pressure differences between the CSF and the venous sinuses. These will be discussed individually below, and mathematical models of CSF dynamics and how they can be used to study these phenomena will be examined.

Production

Determination of accurate production rates of CSF depended on the development of the indicator dilution technique by Pappenheimer et al. (50, 51, 25). In this technique, similar to that used in renal physiology, an indicator in artificial CSF of known concentration is perfused into the ventricular system and then collected at a distant site (Fig. 2.3). The indicators used must remain within the CSF and not diffuse to any significant degree into the brain. As the indicator is added to the ventricular fluid, it becomes diluted by the continuous production of CSF. When the concentration of the indicator collected at the outflow reaches a steady state, CSF production can be calculated using the formula:

$$V_f = V_i \times \frac{C_i - C_o}{C_o} \qquad \text{(eq. 1)}$$

where V_f is the CSF formation rate, V_i is the inflow rate of the indicator, C_i is the concentration of indicator at the inflow, and C_o is the concentration at the outflow. By varying the height of the outflow container, Pappenheimer et al. found little effect of pressure on the rate of CSF formation. Many investigators have used this technique to determine the rate of CSF production in a variety of experimental animals (33, 54). For instance, Rubin et al (61) applied it to determine CSF production in humans. They studied 11 patients with central nervous system (CNS) neoplasms and found that CSF production averaged 0.37 ml/min and was unaffected by intracranial pressure (ICP). Cutler et al (10) applied similar techniques to a group of 12 children with either subacute sclerosing panencephalitis or pontine gliomas and found a mean rate of CSF production of 0.35 ml/min with a standard error of 0.02 ml/min. Lorenzo et al (32) used the method to determine the rate of CSF formation in human hydrocephalus of various etiologies. The mean formation rate was 0.30 ± .02 ml/min, and was also relatively independent of ICP changes. Other techniques have been developed to estimate CSF production rates, but the Pappenheimer technique remains the method by which the others are judged.

The only known condition associated with increased CSF production causing hydrocephalus is found in some patients with choroid plexus papillomas. It was argued for many years that this in fact occurred and by using a ventricular perfusion technique Eisenberg et al. (20) documented a four-fold increase in CSF production in a child with choroid plexus papilloma. Milhorat et al. (47) recorded a preoperative CSF formation rate of 1.05 ml/min and a 5 fold decrease postoperatively in a child with choroid plexus papilloma. Ventricular enlargement in dogs subjected to intraventricular infusions of artificial CSF was recently documented (58), supporting the hypothesis that over-production of CSF can cause hydrocephalus.

Alterations in CSF production rates are less important in other conditions affecting CSF dynamics. ICP is far more dependent upon cerebral hemodynamics than on the rate of CSF production. The reduction of CSF production by one third would decrease the ICP by only 1.5 cm H_2O (10). This may explain why acetazolamide, which reduces CSF production, is minimally effective in the treatment of hydrocephalus.

Choroid Plexus Pulsations

Bering (5) has proposed that CSF is circulated actively by the choroid plexus and that these structures are necessary for the development of hydrocephalus. The pumping force is generated as the choroid plexus fills with blood with each arterial pulsation. Expanding on Dandy's (11) original work in dogs made hydrocephalic with kaolin, Bering performed unilateral choroid plexectomy on dogs and then induced hydrocephalus with kaolin, which blocks the outflow foramina of the fourth ventricle. He found that the ventricle with the remaining choroid plexus became enlarged, whereas the one without remained small. He concluded that back pressure from obstruction to the outlet foramina of the fourth ventricle by kaolin could not be the cause of ventricular dilatation because only one ventricle became enlarged, and that the choroid plexus pressure wave was necessary for the development of the ipsilateral ventriculomegaly.

Milhorat (41) found contradictory results in experiments on rhesus monkeys and concluded that the choroid plexus was not necessary for hydrocephalus to develop. In his experiments, hydrocephalus developed in bilateral plexectomized animals with balloon obstruction of the fourth ventricle, and in unilateral plexectomized animals both ventricles dilated. DiRocco et al. (16) reported inducing hydrocephalus by increasing the amplitude of the intraventricular CSF pulsations without elevating the mean CSF pressure. They instilled a latex balloon in the lateral ventricle of lambs and inflated and deflated the balloon synchronously with the physiological choroidal pulse. Ventricular dilatation occurred in animals whose choroidal pulsations were continuous as well as intermittent, 2 hours every other day. They concluded that abnormally high intraventricular CSF pressure oscillation may be the cause of ventricular dilatation seen in normal-pressure hydrocephalus. These conflicting reports show that the role of choroidal pulsation in CSF circulation and production of hydrocephalus is unclear, but may be important in some pathological conditions such as normal-pressure hydrocephalus.

Resistance

After the CSF is produced, it circulates through a series of conduits and is ultimately absorbed. Possible areas of increased resistance to the flow of CSF would include the foramen of Monro, aqueduct of Sylvius, foramina of Luschka and Magendie, and the arachnoid villi. Resistance across them has been difficult to measure, primarily because of presumed small pressure differentials and the slow flow of the CSF through the pathways, necessitating

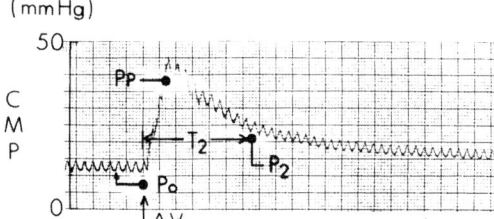

(mmHg)

Figure 2.4. Diagram of the pressure response at the cisterna magna after a bolus injection (ΔV) over time. (Reprinted with permission from A. Marmarou, K. Shulman, J. LaMorgese, Compartmental analysis of compliance and outflow resistance of the cerebrospinal fluid system. J. Neurosurg. *43*:523–534, 1975.)

study of total outflow resistance. Outflow resistance can be estimated using steady state methods or bolus infusions. Under steady state conditions, resistance can be calculated using the equation resistance = pressure change/flow, or by calculating the slope of the line drawn when plotting pressure against absorption. The upper limit of normal using this method is 180 mm saline ml/min (10).

Using this method Martins (37) calculated resistance in 29 patients with a variety of intracranial pathologies. Although resistance was increased to greater than normal in many conditions considered to impede CSF drainage, this was not always the case. Marmarou et al (35) devised a formula to calculate resistance by performing rapid injections of volumes of saline and recording the resultant pressure rise and the time needed for return to baseline. Using this method, outflow resistance can be calculated by the formula:

$$R_o = \frac{t_2 \cdot P_o}{PVI \times \log_{10}\left[\frac{P_2 \cdot P_p - P_o}{P_p \cdot P_2 - P_o}\right]} \quad \text{(eq. 2)}$$

where P_o is initial pressure prior to volume injection, P_p is peak pressure induced by volume injection, P_2 is the instantaneous pressure at an elapsed time (T_2) of the recovery slope, and t_2 is the elapsed time from the instant of volume injection to the point at which P_2 is determined. PVI is an expression of cerebral compliance (Fig. 2.4). Several authors who compared the bolus method with the constant infusion method in determining resistance found that the bolus method underestimated resistance when compared to the steady state method (21, 69). However, both methods give consistent results and are clinically applicable.

Using a constant-pressure infusion method Ekstedt (22) has argued that conductance, the inverse of resistance, is a more appropriate term to use when discussing CSF hydrodynamics.

Absorption

Absorption can also be studied using the Pappenheimer indicator dilution technique (50, 51, 25). The rate of bulk absorption can be calculated using the formula,

$$V_a = \frac{V_i C_i - V_o C_o}{C_o} \quad \text{(eq. 3)}$$

where V_a is the absorption rate, V_i is the inflow perfusion rate, V_o is the outflow rate, C_i is the concentration of the inflow, and C_o is the concentration of the outflow, by perfusing the ventricular system in a manner similar to that for calculating formation rates. Studies of absorption using this technique have revealed that absorption rates increase linearly with increasing pressure (25, 10, 32). Cutler et al. (10) studied formation and absorption over a wide range of pressures (Fig. 2.5). Formation was independent of pressure whereas absorption increased linearly with pressures above 68 mm H_2O. Below 68 mm H_2O no absorption occurred, suggesting an intrinsic resistance that must be overcome. At 112 mm H_2O, formation and absorption rates are equal, presumably representing the average physiological pressure. These two processes act in concert to control CSF pressure within the normal range.

Lorenzo et al. (32) studied absorption in hydrocephalus and described 2 types of absorption defects. In the first patient group, absorption did not begin until pressures much higher than normal were established; with increasing ICP, the absorption rate was about the same as for normal patients. The second group began to absorb CSF at about the same pressure as normal patients, with increasing pressure the absorption rate was less than for normal patients. Some patients could not be put into either group.

Although the Pappenheimer technique is reproducible and accurate, it has 2 drawbacks. Because a steady state of indicator must be obtained in the outflow before calculations can be made, it is very time-consuming, and because it requires ventricular catheters, it is invasive.

Other methods without these disadvantages have been developed. Katzman et al (29) developed a constant infusion test where saline is infused into the lumbar subarachnoid space at a

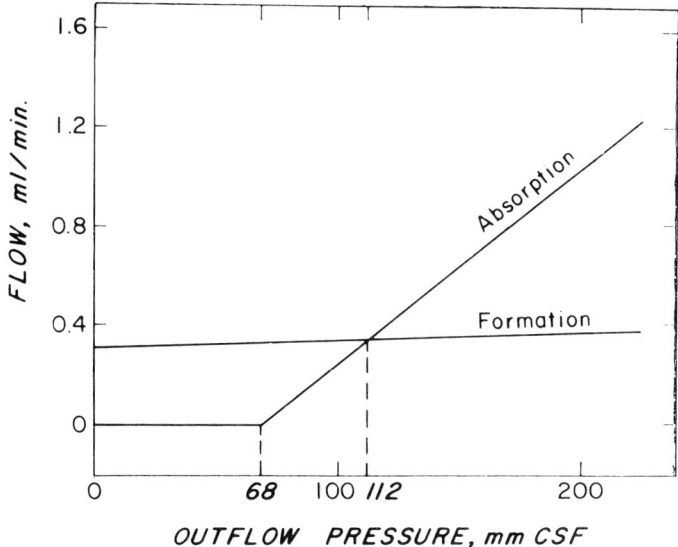

Figure 2.5.   Diagram of CSF formation and absorption over a range of outflow pressures. (Reprinted with permission from R.W.P. Cutler, L. Page, J. Galicich, G.V. Watters, Formation and absorption of cerebrospinal fluid in man. Brain: *91*:707–720, 1968.)

constant rate, and the pressure change is measured by using a manometer. It is assumed that CSF formation is independent of CSF pressure (10, 20, 32). There is no outflow cannula so all the infused fluid will either distend the subarachnoid space or be absorbed into the bloodstream. In normal subjects, as the infusion continues, the CSF pressure rises and eventually plateaus, usually within 40-60 minutes. At steady state, infusion rate plus production is equal to absorption. Production is assumed to be approximately 0.35 ml/min (10). An infusion rate of 0.76 ml/min was chosen as one well tolerated by normal patients with small elevations in CSF pressure. Applying this test to various clinical situations, the authors found that abnormal responses resulted in much higher pressure elevations for a given infusion rate than in normal patients (27). They concluded that the test was useful in evaluating pediatric patients with possible arrested hydrocephalus or shunt malfunction, and in adult patients with communicating hydrocephalus. Although the constant infusion test has the advantage of being relatively noninvasive, it is time-consuming, requiring several hours to obtain a pressure equilibrium.

Ekstedt (21) and Portnoy et al. (56, 57) have described a method of constant pressure CSF infusion using lumbar needles for infusion, recording pressure, and collecting CSF. First a resting pressure is determined, and then various pressures set above and below the resting pressure and the rate of CSF infusion or drainage is established. This method's main advantage over the others is the rapidity with which a constant pressure-constant flow steady state can be reached, making it possible to determine several values in the same subject.

Sagittal Sinus Pressure

That CSF circulation is governed by the physics of bulk flow and is not just a diffusion or secretion has been well established. Therefore, flow is proportional to the pressure gradient between the subarachnoid space and the dural sinuses according to the equation,

$$F = \frac{P_1 - P_2}{R} \qquad \text{(eq. 4)}$$

where F is flow, P_1 is subarachnoid pressure, P_2 is dural sinus pressure, and R is the resistance to absorption. Flow across the arachnoid villi or absorption is dependent upon this pressure gradient. The normal pressure difference in humans is approximately 30-40 mm H_2O, similar to the pressure gradient in experimental animals (12, 63, 65). If the pressure gradient is lost, absorption into the superior sagittal sinus becomes zero.

The relation between ICP and dural sinus pressure is unclear. Attempts to induce hydrocephalus in animals by blocking the major dural venous sinuses have been largely unsuccessful, although Bering et al. (4) were able to produce hydrocephalus in dogs by blocking the cephalic venous drainage in the neck. In adult humans, dural sinus blockage is associated with the symptom of pseudotumor cerebri; however, Kinal (30) reported 4 hydrocephalic children with abnormal dural sinus venography and suggested a causal relationship. Recently, achondroplastic dwarfs with hydrocephalus have been reported to have blockage to venous outflow at the jugular foramen (52). These data suggest that blockage of the dural sinuses in adults with nondistensible skulls leads to intracranial hypertension without hydrocephalus, whereas in children with open sutures, ventricular dilatation occurs.

Elevation of ICP has resulted in inconsistent changes in sagittal sinus pressure. Reporting on animal studies, Weed and Flexner (71) stated that even profound changes in subarachnoid pressure were unaccompanied by changes in superior sagittal sinus pressure. Bedford (3) found a consistent fall in sagittal sinus pressure with increases of subarachnoid pressure to 500 mm H_2O, and Wright (74) reported an initial rise followed by a fall in sagittal sinus pressure with elevated CSF pressure. In humans, Osterholm (49) studied 5 patients with acute neurological deterioration from extraaxial lesions following severe cranial trauma and recorded both elevation in sagittal sinus pressure and partial obstruction of the sinus drainage on venography. Martins et al. (38) noted inconsistent findings in 12 patients with brain tumor, the majority showing no rise in sagittal sinus pressure with elevated ICA, but several showing elevations.

In hydrocephalus in both experimental animals and humans, the pressure differential that normally exists between the sagittal sinus and CSF is in many cases lost. When Shulman et al. (65) studied normal dogs and dogs made hydrocephalic with kaolin, they found that in normal dogs, CSF pressure was greater than sagittal sinus pressure, which is greater than torcular pressure. However, in hydrocephalic dogs, the mean CSF pressure was approximately equal to sagittal sinus pressure, and both were greater than torcular pressure. (In dogs the torcular is encased in bone.) Shulman et al. postulated a partial collapse of the sagittal sinus to account for the elevated pressure in hydrocephalus. In another study of 15 hydrocephalic patients with various etiologies Shulman et al. (66) found a consistent pressure elevation within the sagittal sinus. Sinograms performed on several of these children revealed compression of the sinuses near the point of exit from the skull. Sainte-Rose et al. (63) studied 20 hydrocephalic infants and children with increased sagittal sinus pressure. In most patients without anatomical interruption of the sinus, CSF withdrawals induced a simultaneous decrease of ICP and sagittal sinus pressure. In several patients with achondroplasia or craniostenosis and anatomical blockage of the sinus, CSF withdrawal caused lowering of ICP but not sagittal sinus pressure. On one of these latter children, vein bypass was performed around the obstruction and ventricular size decreased without the need for a ventricular shunt. Norrell et al. (48) recorded a less constant elevation in sagittal sinus pressure in 30 hydrocephalic children in whom an elevation occurred much more frequently in those patients with myelomeningocele than in others. In many children with myelomeningocele the dural sinuses have an abnormal configuration. Norrell's data suggest that some types of hydrocephalus cause deformation of the sinus drainage, increasing the resistance to flow. This increased resistance elevates the pressure in the sagittal sinus, thereby decreasing or eliminating the pressure differential across the arachnoid villi necessary for CSF absorption.

TOWARD A MATHEMATICAL MODEL OF CSF DYNAMICS

To understand the pathophysiology of hydrocephalus in its various forms and other abnormalities of production and absorption of CSF, a mathematical model incorporating all factors that interact to control CSF production and absorption, as well as factors within the brain that affect regulation of the volume of the cerebral ventricles, would be very helpful. Several such models have been constructed based on sound physiological and mathematical principles. Few, however, have been validated by physiological data (1, 24, 34, 36, 59, 67, 68). A mathematical model lending itself to a computer simulation that could be validated by physiological studies would be a powerful tool for studying the pathophysiology of hydrocephalus.

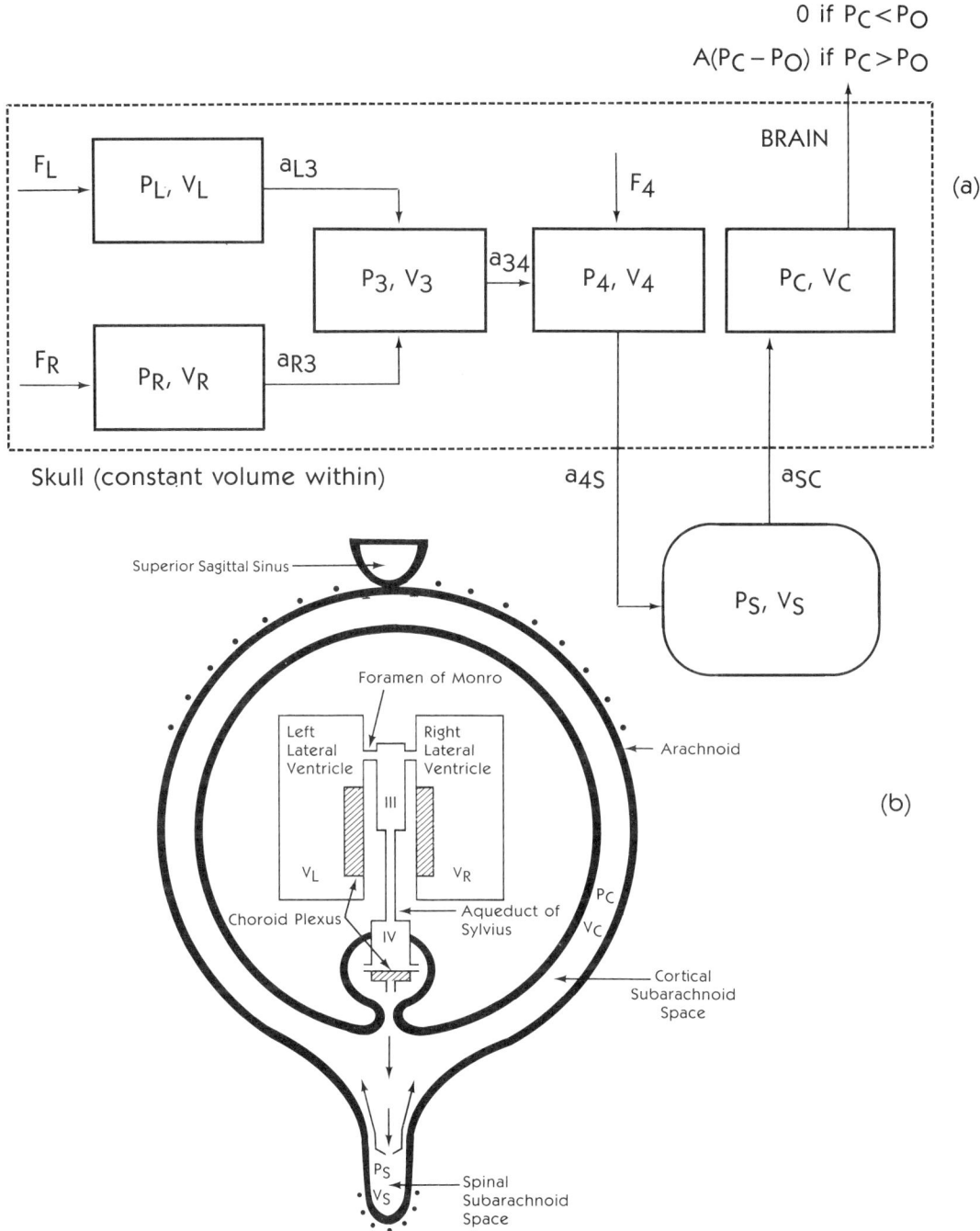

Figure 2.6. Diagrammatic and schematic representation of a multicompartmental model of ventricular volume and cerebrospinal fluid flow (Reprinted with permission from H.L. Rekate *et al.*, The application of mathematical modeling to hydrocephalus research. In: *Concepts in Pediatric Neurosurgery*, Vol. 8., edited by A.E. Marlin, pp. 1–14, Basel, Karger Inc. 1988.

Building on concepts proposed by Marmarou and later described by Spertell, such a mathematical model has been developed (36, 68). Based on principles of fluid dynamics and using a systems engineering approach, the model employs a multiple compartment arrangement described in Fig. 2.6. The assumptions on which the model is based include the following:

1. The volume of the lateral ventricles, third ventricle, fourth ventricle, cortical subarachnoid space, and brain is fixed by the rigid skull. Mathematically, this is represented as

$$V_R + V_L + V_{III} + V_{IV} + V_{CSAS} + V_B = \text{constant} \quad \text{(eq. 5)}$$

where V_x equals the volume of the compartments. Another way of looking at this is to say that any change in one compartment must be compensated for by a change in the volume of the other compartments—mathematically represented as

$$\frac{dV_L}{dT} + \frac{dV_R}{dT} + \frac{dV_{III}}{dT} + \frac{dV_{IV}}{dT} + \frac{dV_{CSAS}}{dT} + \frac{dV_B}{dT} = 0 \quad \text{(eq. 6)}$$

2. The relatively large volume of the spinal subarachnoid space lies outside the skull's constraint.
3. Just as water flows downhill, CSF flows from higher states of energy to lower states, and its flow can be represented mathematically by formulae analogous to the electrical formula

$$V = IR \quad \text{(eq. 7)}$$

where V is the difference in energy state (i.e., height of a column of liquid), I is the flow rate (in this model, in ml/min), and R is the resistance in torr/ml/min. In this model, therefore, the flow across the left foramen of Monro is represented as

$$\frac{dV_L}{dT} = F_L - \alpha_{L, III} (P_L - P_{III}) \quad \text{(eq. 8)}$$

where $\frac{dV_L}{dT}$ is the change in volume with respect to time of the left lateral ventricles, F_L is the formation rate of cerebrospinal fluid within the left lateral ventricles, P is the pressure within the compartment in question and α connotes conductance, which is the inverse of resistance.

4. The final major assumption of this model is that the brain itself has both intrinsic characteristics related to its blood volume and intrinsic viscoelastic characteristics. These are important in determining to what extent energy added to the system causes an increase in ventricular size or ICP.

The construction and utility of a mathematical model are described elsewhere (59). Review of the assumptions and principles involved in the design of such a model can add to our understanding of the pathophysiology of hydrocephalus.

REFERENCES

1. Agarwal, G., Berman, B., Stark L., *et al.* A lumped parameter model of the cerebrospinal fluid system. IEEE Trans. Biomed. Eng. *1:*45–53, 1969.
2. Alksne, J.F. and Lovings, E.T. Functional ultrastructure of the arachnoid villus. Arch. Neurol. *27:*371–377, 1972.
3. Bedford, T.H.B. The effect of variations in the subarachnoid pressure on the venous pressure in the superior longitudinal sinus and in the torcular of the dog. J. Physiol. *101:*362–368, 1942.
4. Bering, E.A. Jr. and Salibi, B. Production of hydrocephalus by increased cephalic-venous pressure. Arch. Neurol. & Psychiat. *81:*693–698, 1959.
5. Bering, E.A. Jr. Circulation of the cerebrospinal fluid. Demonstration of the choroid plexuses as the generator of the force for flow of fluid and ventricular enlargement. J. Neurosurg. *19:*405–413, 1962.
6. Brightman, M.W. The intracerebral movement of proteins injected into blood and cerebrospinal fluid of mice. Prog. Brain Res. *29:*19–40, 1968.
7. Casley-Smith, J.R., Földi-Börcsök, E., and Földi, M. The prelymphatic pathways of the brain as revealed by cervical lymphatic obstruction and the passage of particles. Br. J. Exp. Pathol. *57:*179–188, 1976.
8. Cserr, H.F. Physiology of the choroid plexus. Physiol. Rev. *51(2):*273–331, 1971.
9. Cserr, H.F, Cooper, D.N., Suri, P.K., *et al.* Efflux of radiolabeled polyethylene glycols and albumin from rat brain. Am. J. Physiol. *240:*F319–F328, 1981.
10. Cutler, R.W.P., Page, L., Galicich, J., *et al.* Formation and absorption of cerebrospinal fluid in man. Brain *91:*707–720, 1968.
11. Dandy, W.E. Experimental hydrocephalus. Ann. Surg. *70(2):*129–142, 1919.
12. D'Avella, D., Greenberg, R.P., Mingrino, S., *et al.* Alterations in ventricular size and intracranial pressure caused by sagittal sinus pathology in man. J. Neurosurg. *53:*656–661, 1980.
13. Davidoff, L.M. Hydrocephalus, and hydrocephalus with meningocele; their treatment by choroid plexectomy. Surg. Clin. North Am. *28:*416–431, 1948.
14. Davson, H., Domer, F.R., and Hollingsworth, J.R. The mechanism of drainage of the cerebrospinal fluid. Brain *96:*329–336, 1973.
15. DiRocco, C., DiTrapani, G., Pettorossi, V.E., *et al.* On the pathology of experimental hydrocephalus induced by artificial increase in endoventricular CSF pulse pressure. Childs Brain *5:*81–95, 1979.
16. Dorhmann, G.J. and Bucy, P.C. Human choroid plexus: a light and electron microscopic study. J. Neurosurg. *33:*506–516, 1970.
17. Dohrmann, G.J. The choroid plexus in experimental hydrocephalus. A light and electron microscopic study in normal, hydrocephalic, and shunted hydrocephalic dogs. J. Neurosurg. *34:*56–69, 1971.

18. Eisenberg, H.M., McLennan, J.E., and Welch, K. Ventricular perfusion in cats with kaolin-induced hydrocephalus. J. Neurosurg. *41*:20–28, 1974.

19. Eisenberg, H.M., McComb, J.G., and Lorenzo, A.V. Cerebrospinal fluid overproduction and hydrocephalus associated with choroid plexus papilloma. J. Neurosurg. *40*:381–385, 1974.

20. Ekstedt, J. CSF hydrodynamic studies in man. 1. Method of constant pressure CSF infusion. J. Neurol. Neurosurg. Psychiatry *40*:105–119, 1977.

21. Ekstedt, J. CSF hydrodynamic studies in man. 2. Normal hydrodynamic variables related to CSF pressure and flow. J. Neurol. Neurosurg. Psychiatry *41*:345–353, 1978.

22. Földi, M., Csillik, B., and Zoltan, O.T. Lymphatic drainage of the brain. Experientia *24*:1283–1287, 1968.

23. Guinane, J.E. An equivalent circuit analysis of cerebrospinal fluid hydrodynamics. Am. J. Physiol. *223*:425–430, 1972.

24. Heisey, S.R., Held, D., and Pappenheimer, J.R. Bulk flow and diffusion in the cerebrospinal fluid system of the goat. Am. J. Physiol. *203*:775–781, 1962.

25. Hiratsuka, H., Tabata, H., Tsuruoka, S., et al. Evaluation of periventricular hypodensity in experimental hydrocephalus by metrizamide CT ventriculography. J. Neurosurg. *56*:235–240, 1982.

26. Hussey, F., Schanzer, B., and Katzman, R. A simple constant-infusion manometric test for measurement of CSF absorption. II. Clinical studies. Neurology *20*:665–680, 1970.

27. Jackson, R.T., Tigges, J., and Arnold, W. Subarachnoid space of the CNS, nasal mucosa, and lymphatic system. Arch. Otolaryngol. *105*:180–184, 1979.

28. Katzman, R. and Hussey, F. A simple constant-infusion manometric test for measurement of CSF absorption. 1. Rationale and method. Neurology *20*:534–544, 1970.

29. Kinal, M.E. Hydrocephalus and the dural venous sinuses. J. Neurosurg. *19*:195–201, 1962.

30. Kosteljanetz, M. Resistance to outflow of cerebrospinal fluid determined by bolus injection technique and constant rate steady state infusion in humans. Neurosurgery *16*:336–340, 1985.

31. Lorenzo, A.V., Page, L.K., and Watters, G.V. Relationship between cerebrospinal fluid formation, absorption and pressure in human hydrocephalus. Brain *93*:679–692, 1970.

32. Lux, W.E., Jr. and Fenstermacher, J.D. Cerebrospinal fluid formation in ventricles and spinal subarachnoid space of the rhesus monkey. J. Neurosurg. *42*:674–678, 1975.

33. Marmarou, A. *A theoretical model and experimental evaluation of the cerebrospinal fluid system.* Ph.D. thesis, Drexel University, pp 1–142, 1973.

34. Marmarou, A., Shulman, K., and LaMorgese, J. Compartmental analysis of compliance and outflow resistance of the cerebrospinal fluid system. J. Neurosurg. *43*:523–534, 1975.

35. Marmarou, A., Shulman, K., and Rosende, R. A nonlinear analysis of the cerebrospinal fluid system and intracranial pressure dynamics. J. Neurosurg. *48*:332–334, 1978.

36. Martins, A.N. Resistance to drainage of cerebrospinal fluid: Clinical measurement and significance. J. Neurol. Neurosurg. Psychiatry *36*:313–318, 1973.

37. Martins, A.N., Kobrine, A.I., and Larsen, D.F. Pressure in the sagittal sinus during intracranial hypertension in man. J. Neurosurg. *40*:603–608, 1974.

38. McComb, J.G., Davson, H., and Hollingsworth, J.R. Attempted separation of blood-brain and blood-cerebrospinal fluid barriers in the rabbit. Exp. Eye Res. *25(Suppl)*:333–343, 1977.

39. McComb, J.G. Review article: Recent research into the nature of cerebrospinal fluid formation and absorption. J. Neurosurg. *59*:369–383, 1983.

40. Milhorat, T.H. Choroid plexus and cerebrospinal fluid production. Science *166*:1514–1516, 1969.

41. Milhorat, T.H., Mosher, M.B., Hammock, M.K., et al. Evidence for choroid plexus absorption in hydrocephalus. N. Engl. J. Med. *283(6)*:286–289, 1970.

42. Milhorat, T.H., Hammock, M.K., Fenstermacher, J.D., et al. Cerebrospinal fluid production by the choroid plexus and brain (abstract). Science *173*:330–332, 1971.

43. Milhorat, T.H. Failure of choroid plexectomy as treatment for hydrocephalus. Surg. Gynecol. Obst. *139*:505–508, 1974.

44. Milhorat, T.H. The third circulation revisited. J. Neurosurg. *42*:628–645, 1975.

45. Milhorat, T.H., Hammock, M.K., Chien, T., et al. Normal rate of cerebrospinal fluid formation five years after bilateral choroid plexectomy: Case report. J. Neurosurg. *44*:735–739, 1976.

46. Milhorat, T.H., Hammock, M.K., Davis, D.A., et al. Choroid plexus papilloma 1. Proof of cerebrospinal fluid overproduction. Child's Brain *2*:273–289, 1976.

47. Norrell, H., Wilson, C., Howieson, J., et al. Venous factors in infantile hydrocephalus. J. Neurosurg. *31*:561–569, 1969.

48. Osterholm, J.L. Reaction of the cerebral venous sinus system to acute intracranial hypertension. J. Neurosurg. *32*:654–659, 1970.

49. Pappenheimer, J.R., Heisey, S.R., and Jordan, E.F. Active transport of Diodrast and phenolsulfonphthalein from cerebrospinal fluid to blood. Am. J. Physiol. *200(1)*:1–10, 1961.

50. Pappenheimer, J.R., Heisey, S.R., Jordan, E.F., et al. Perfusion of the cerebral ventricular system in unanesthetized goats. Am. J. Physiol. *203*:763–774, 1962.

51. Pierre-Kahn, A., Hirsch, J.F., Renier, D., et al. Hydrocephalus and achondroplasia. A study of 25 observations. Childs Brain *7*:205–219, 1980.

52. Pollay, M. and Curl, F. Secretion of cerebrospinal fluid by the ventricular ependyma of the rabbit. Am. J. Physiol. *213(4)*:1031–1038, 1967.

53. Pollay, M. Formation of cerebrospinal fluid. Relation of studies of isolated choroid plexus to the standing gradient hypothesis. Neurosurg. *42*:665–673, 1975.

54. Pollay, M., Hisey, B., Reynolds, E., et al. Choroid plexus Na^+/K^+-activated adenosine triphosphatase and cerebrospinal fluid formation. Neurosurgery *17(5)*:768–772, 1985.

55. Portnoy, H.D. and Croissant, P.D. A practical method for measuring hydrodynamics of cerebrospinal fluid. Surg. Neurol. *5*:273–277, 1976.

56. Portnoy, H.D., and Croissant, P.D. Pre- and postoperative cerebrospinal fluid absorption studies in patients with myelomeningocele shunted for hydrocephalus. Childs Brain *4:*47–64, 1978.

57. Rekate, H.L., Erwood, S., Brodkey, J.A., *et al.* Etiology of ventriculomegaly in choroid plexus papilloma. Pediat. Neurosci. *12:*196–201, 1985-86.

58. Rekate, H.L., Williams, F., Chizeck, H.J., *et al.* The application of mathematical modeling to hydrocephalus research. In *Concepts in Pediatric Neurosurgery, Vol 8.,* edited by A.E. Marlin, Basel, Karger, pp. 1–14, 1988.

59. Rosenberg, G.A., Kyner, W.T., and Estrada, E. Bulk flow of brain interstitial fluid under normal and hyperosmolar conditions. Am. J. Physiol. *238:*F42–F49, 1980.

60. Rubin, R.C., Henderson, E.S., Ommaya, A.K., *et al.* The production of cerebrospinal fluid in man and its modification by acetazolamide. J. Neurosurg. *25:*430–436, 1966.

61. Sahar, A. Choroidal origin of cerebrospinal fluid. Isr. J. Med. Sci. *8(5):*594–596, 1972.

62. Sainte-Rose, C., LaCombe, J., Pierre-Kahn, A., *et al.* Intracranial venous sinus hypertension: Cause or consequence of hydrocephalus in infants? J. Neurosurg. *60:*727–736, 1984.

63. Shabo, A.L. and Maxwell, D.S. The morphology of the arachnoid villi: A light and electron microscopic study in the monkey. J. Neurosurg. *29:*451–463, 1968.

64. Shulman, K., Yarnell, P., and Ransohoff, J. Dural sinus pressure in normal and hydrocephalic dogs. Arch. Neurol. *10:*575–580, 1964.

65. Shulman, K. and Ransohoff, J. Sagittal sinus venous pressure in hydrocephalus. J. Neurosurg. *23:*169–173, 1965.

66. Simon, R., Lehman, R., and O'Connor, S. A comparison of pressure-volume models in hydrocephalus. Neurosurgery *15:*694–699, 1984.

67. Spertell, R. The response of brain to transient evaluations in intraventricular pressure. J. Neurol. Sci. *48:*343–352, 1980.

68. Takizawa, H., Gabra-Sanders, T., and Miller, J.D. Validity of measurements of cerebrospinal fluid outflow resistance estimated by the bolus injection method. Neurosurgery *17:*63–66, 1985.

69. Upton, M.L. and Weller, R.O. The morphology of cerebrospinal fluid drainage pathways in human arachnoid granulations. J. Neurosurg. *63:*867–875, 1985.

70. Weed, L.H. and Flexner, L.B. Relations of intracranial pressures. Am. J. Physiol. *105:*266–272, 1933.

71. Welch, K. and Friedman, V. The cerebrospinal fluid valves. Brain *83:*454–469, 1960.

72. Welch, K. Secretion of cerebrospinal fluid by choroid plexus of the rabbit. Am. J. Physiol. *205*(3):617–624, 1963.

73. Wright, R.D. Experimental observations on increased intracranial pressure. Aust. N.Z. J. Surg. *7:*215–235, 1938.

CHAPTER 3

Radiological Investigation of Pediatric Hydrocephalus

SAMUEL M. WOLPERT, M.D.

INTRODUCTION

Hydrocephalus can be defined as the condition in which the ventricular volume of cerebrospinal fluid (CSF) is abnormally large in relation to the volume of the brain. The cause of the hydrocephalus is an important consideration in patient management. If the hydrocephalus is secondary to blockage of the CSF pathways, the hydrocephalus will be progressive and require active treatment. If the hydrocephalus is secondary to cerebral white matter loss, as may be found in some cases of severe head trauma or dementing processes (e.g., hydrocephalus ex vacuo), the hydrocephalus is usually static and does not require treatment.

No one classification system of hydrocephalus is perfect since often the causes may be classified under more than one heading. The following etiological classification, adopted from Russell (33), will be used in this chapter.

(A) Obstructive
   a) Ventricular blockage (internal—non-communicating)
      1) congenital anomalies
      2) post-inflammatory blockage
      3) post-hemorrhagic blockage
      4) tumors
   b) Cisternal blockage (external—communicating)
      1) congenital anomalies
      2) post-inflammatory blockage
      3) post-hemorrhagic blockage
      4) venous thrombosis
      5) tumors
(B) Non-obstructive
   a) Atrophic process
(C) Functional
   a) Hypersecretion
   b) Impaired absorption

Classification by obstruction site is limited in some patients because the obstruction is at more than one level. Nevertheless, in most cases this classification is useful and practical.

DIAGNOSTIC TESTS

The radiologist's role in patient management when hydrocephalus is suspected is two-fold: firstly, to establish that hydrocephalus is present, and secondly, to determine the cause if possible. Before the advent of computed tomography (CT), the evaluation of the patient with suspected hydrocephalus commenced with a skull roentgenogram, a test that today is usually bypassed although important information could be obtained from it. For instance, in patients with the Chiari II malformation, the skull x-ray reveals luckenschadel, caused by mesodermal dysplasia of the skull, and a low inion. The inion is also low in patients with congenital aqueduct stenosis, and it is high in the Dandy-Walker syndrome and in patients with retrocerebellar arachnoid cysts. After the first year of life other specific skull x-ray findings may help to localize a lesion causing ventricular obstruction, such as solitary intracranial calcifications associated with tumors (e.g., craniopharyngiomas, oligodendrogliomas, pinealomas, choroid plexus papillomas), or focal changes such as sellar enlargement.

The most important management issue is the size of the ventricles, so the diagnostic workup should commence with a cranial ultrasound study, or CT or magnetic resonance imaging (MRI) scan. For the infant patient, ultrasound is a most useful test, not only to establish the presence of hydrocephalus but often to identify the cause. It easily identifies neonatal hemor-

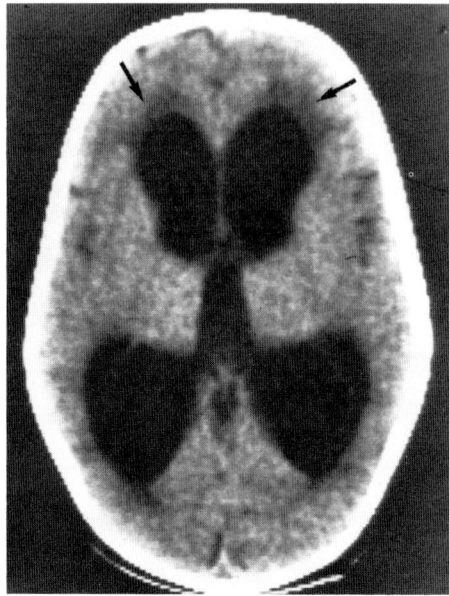

Figure 3.1. Note the symmetrical enlargement of the anterior horns, atria, occipital horns, and third ventricle. The hypodensity seen adjacent to the anterior horns (arrows) is due to trans-ependymal CSF flow.

rhage and can be used to follow the effects of ventricular shunting. Unfortunately, ultrasound does not have the spatial resolution achieved with CT or MRI, which therefore may also be necessary. The relative value of CT and MRI in managing hydrocephalus is the subject of considerable clinical research. On many occasions the choice may be imposed by considerations of availablity and cost rather than diagnostic efficacy. Both CT and MRI can reveal enlargement of the ventricles or cortical subarachnoid spaces, but CT can miss small lesions in the region of the aqueduct or foramen of Monro. MRI can miss calcification, unless it is large and dense. The intravenous administration of a radio-opaque contrast agent with CT is often necessary to precisely delineate most intracranial masses, as the paramagnetic contrast agent Gadolinium-DTPA is often similarly used in MRI.

In the infant the normal mild physiological enlargement of the ventricles may be misdiagnosed as hydrocephalus. The telencephalic basal ganglionic mass is phylogenetically far ahead of the cortex in terms of growth and maturation. At birth and in the weeks immediately before, the cortex may not as yet have caught up with the growth of the deeper structures, creating an impression of large basal ganglia, large lateral ventricles, and a thin cortical mantle. After birth, as the brain matures, the relative size of the frontal horns (Evan's ratio), the interhemispheric and Sylvian fissures, and the third ventricle decrease (28).

Ventricular enlargement (Fig. 3.1) initially occurs at the expense of the immediately adjacent white or gray matter rather than at the expense of the cortex (11). In the neonate generalized lateral ventricular enlargement does not occur equally throughout all regions of the lateral ventricle, in contrast to the more proportional distribution of the enlargement when it occurs at an older age. The earliest sign of neonatal or infantile hydrocephalus is dilatation of the occipital horns and atria of the lateral ventricles followed shortly by blunting of the dorsolateral angles of the ventricles above the caudate nuclei and the thalami (11). There are many theoretical explanations for this phenomenon: discontinuity of the ependyma of the occipital horn throughout the latter half of gestation may promote preferential expansion of the occipital horns; rapid outward growth of the temporal, parietal, and occipital lobes may occur more easily because the parietal bone is relatively free-floating whereas the frontal bone is attached to the skull base; the large mass of choroid plexus in the atria of the lateral ventricles promotes a pulsatile pressure wave that is maximal at the atria; or the white matter surrounding the frontal horns is partially bordered and protected from expansion by the gray matter of the heads of the caudate nuclei (11, 26), whereas the periatrial white matter has no such support (26).

With severe hydrocephalus, diverticuli may project into the paraventricular white matter; this can be detected by CT. Medial atrial diverticuli can herniate through the tentorial incisura to compress the cerebellum (25). A fairly common change in the periventricular white matter in acute hydrocephalus is an increase in its water content due to transependymal flow of CSF from elevated intraventricular pressure (13, 22, 35). Some authors believe that these periventricular tissue changes do not depend upon elevation of the intracranial pressure (ICP) but are simply due to an augmentation of the ventricular pulse pressure (5). The increase in the fluid content of the white matter is seen on CT as areas of periventricular hypodensity (Figs. 3.1, 3.2, 3.3), and on MRI as an in-

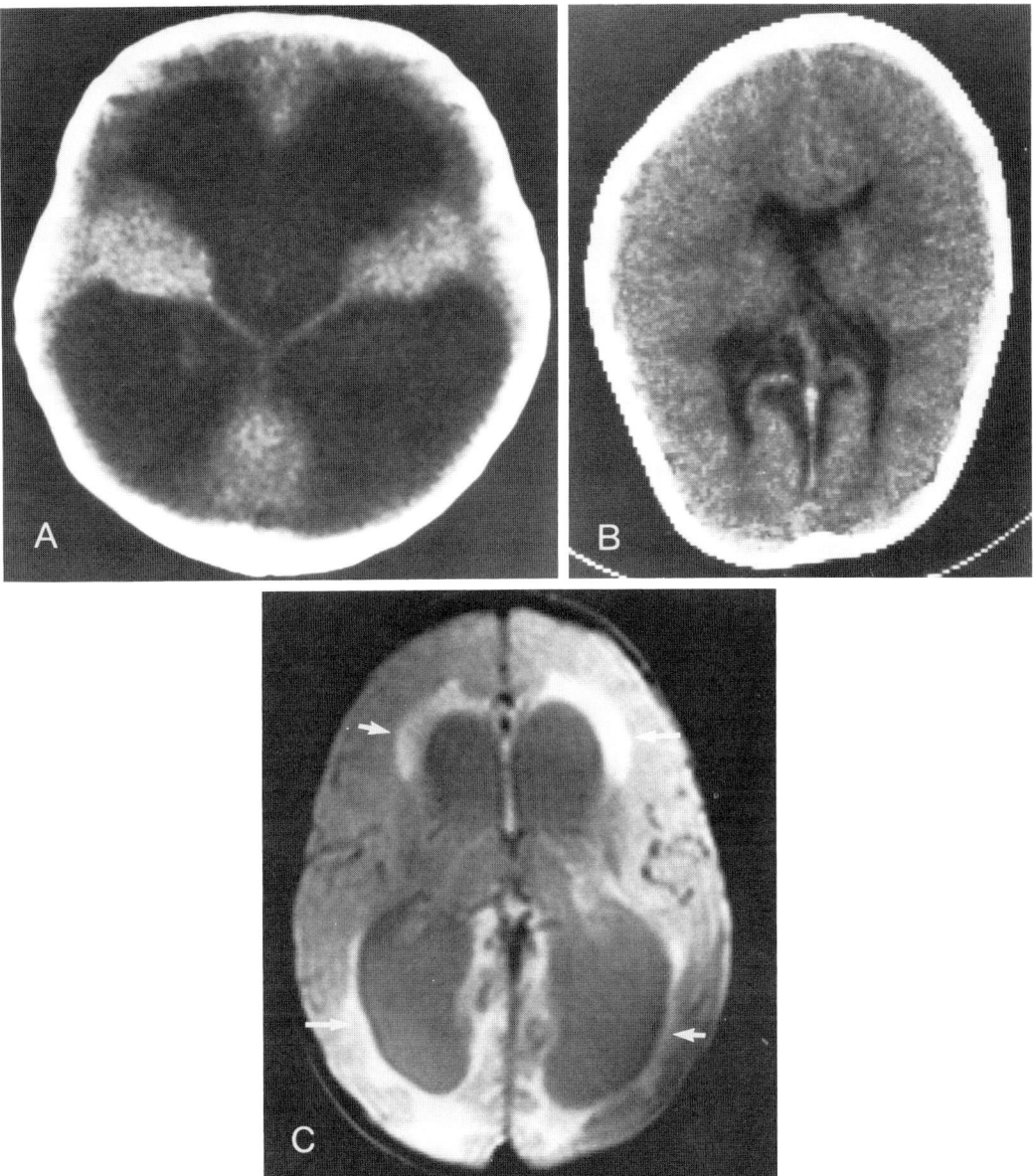

Figure 3.2. *A.* An axial CT scan demonstrates massive enlargement of the lateral ventricular system and third ventricle due to aqueduct stenosis. *B.* Following shunting of the lateral ventricles, marked bulk recovery of the brain ensued at 18 months postshunting. *C.* Axial plane MR, T2-weighted scan demonstrates large lateral ventricles and periventricular hyperintensity (arrows) signifying transependymal CSF flow. Note that the signal intensity is higher than that of the adjacent ventricles, indicating that the extraventricular fluid contains high protein, or that gliosis is associated.

crease in the T1 and T2 values in the white matter (Fig. 3.2c). Characteristically, the abnormality is first seen at the ventricular-white matter junctions. The portions of the ventricular margins that are adjacent to the gray matter of the caudate and thalamus remain sharp until the hydrocephalus becomes longstanding (24).

The fluid lies in the extracellular space, which may be increased by 30% or more (19). Serial CT density measurements after intraventricular administration of a water-soluble contrast medium show progressive increase in the density of the periventricular lucent zone as the opacified intraventricular CSF passes into the per-

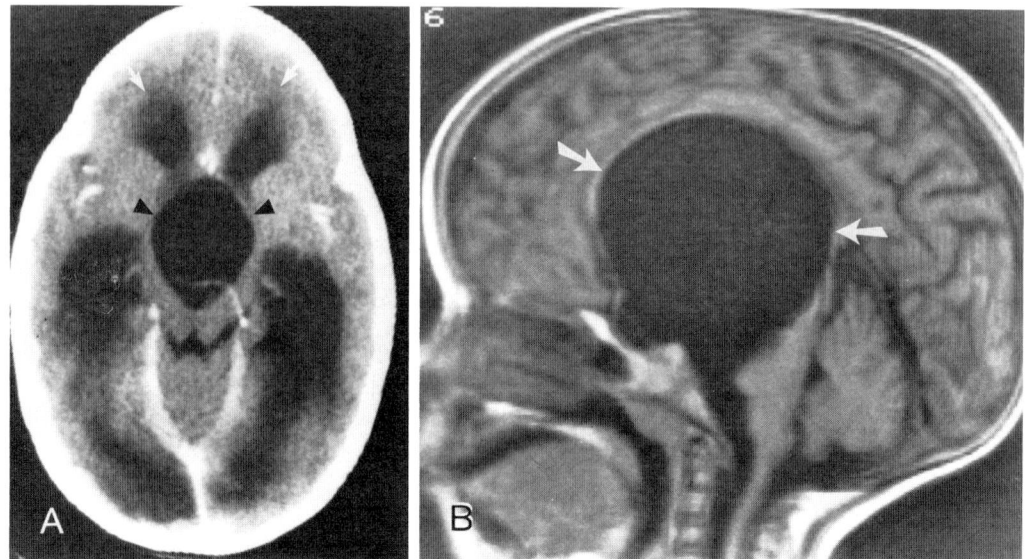

Figure 3.3. *A.* An axial contrast-enhanced CT scan shows massive enlargement of the suprasellar cistern (arrowheads) and hydrocephalus. Note the periventricular hypodensity indicative of transependymal CSF flow (arrows). *B.* Sagittal-plane MR demonstrates a massive suprasellar arachnoid cyst (arrows) obliterating the basal cisterns and third ventricle. The midbrain is displaced posteriorly. (Case courtesy Steven Smith, M.D., Albany, N.Y.).

iventricular space (9, 12). Axonal and myelin destruction can also occur with the increase in the brain's water content (37).

CSF in the parenchyma, indicative of interstitial flow, does not necessarily indicate absorption. The ependymal surface offers essentially no barrier to water (36). The extracellular space, which amounts to 15% of the brain volume, readily allows fluid flow in the parenchyma (20). The flow occurs under normal physiological conditions, and the velocity and direction respond to changes in hydrostatic and osmotic pressure gradients (30, 31). Similarly, the CSF in the subarachnoid spaces may readily penetrate the cerebral parenchyma (6). Evidence thus supports the contention that the brain, rather than absorbing CSF, is acting as a conduit for CSF to move from the ventricles to the subarachnoid space or into the perilymphatic channels of the blood vessels (20).

Following ventricular shunting the periventricular abnormalities resolve (1) and the periventricular white matter recovers its bulk to a considerable degree (Fig. 3.2) (8). Much of the recovery is seen within the first week—indeed, the first day—after shunting (34). To explain this phenomenon, Penn and Bacus (29) suggest brain/water shifts—*i.e.*, a decrease in extracellular fluid in hydrocephalus and an increase in the extracellular fluid following shunting.

However, as mentioned above, there is considerable evidence that the extracellular fluid does not decrease but rather increases with hydrocephalus. Others have noted that after ventricular shunting of hydrocephalic cats the perivascular beds (particularly the large cortical veins) increase and the Virchow-Robin spaces become abnormally dilated (27).

If CSF overdrainage through excessive shunting occurs, the ventricles may collapse around the shunt in the "slit ventricles" syndrome (27). Some of these patients then show decreased transependymal CSF movement into the brain and decreased intracranial compliance. With subsequent shunt obstruction, the ventricles' capacity to expand is lost, and the patient may immediately demonstrate signs of elevated intracranial pressure without ventriculomegaly.

INTERNAL OBSTRUCTIVE HYDROCEPHALUS

Congenital Anomalies

Aqueduct Stenosis

Different conditions affecting the aqueduct may all cause obstructive hydrocephalus. The aqueduct may be congenitally stenosed or "forked," having multiple blind out-pouchings without patency. The aqueduct is invariably visualized in the normal midline sagittal MRI scan (Fig. 3.4), which therefore is an excellent image for diagnosing aqueduct stenosis. Aqueduct stenosis is frequently found in association with the Chiari II malformation where the stenosis is probably due to compression, dorsal displacement, and angulation of the aqueduct by the enlarged atria and bodies of the lateral ventricles (Fig. 3.5). Both CT and MRI can reveal the Arnold-Chiari malformation. However, the excellent spatial resolution of high-field MRI demonstrates not only the herniated hind-brain but also the patency of the aqueduct and other associated cerebral malformations. A region of increased periaqueductal signal is often seen on axial T2 weighted scans in normal patients (Fig. 3.4C). This appearance

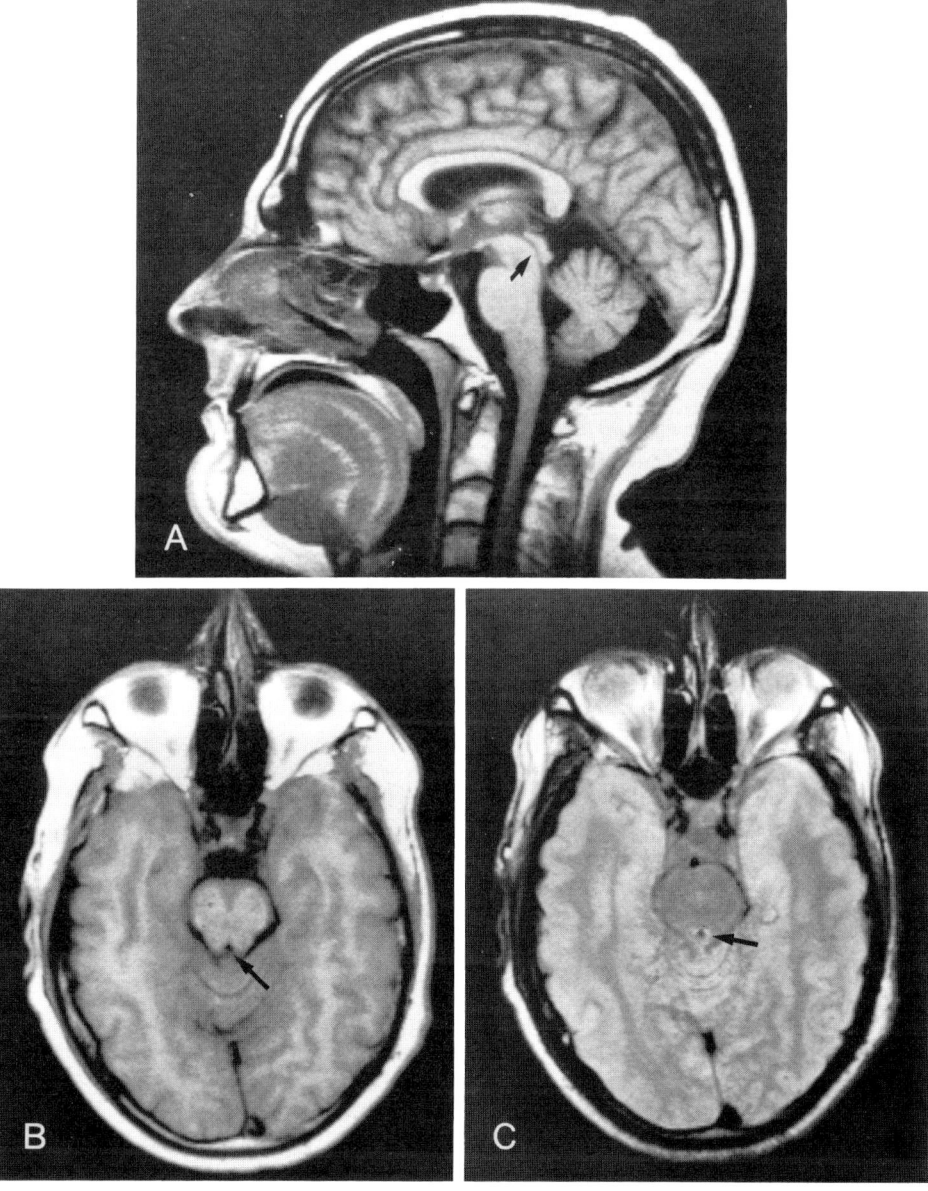

Figure 3.4. *A.* A sagittal plane T1-weighted scan demonstrates a normal patent aqueduct. *B.* The aqueduct (arrow) is also seen on axial spin density and *C.* T2-weighted scans. On the latter, note the periaqueductal high density (arrow), which is a normal finding.

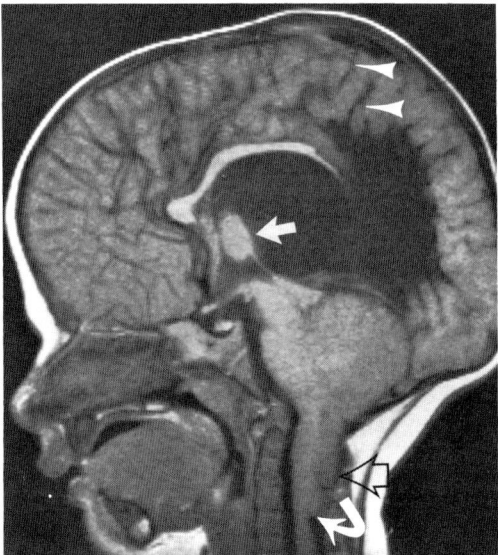

Figure 3.5. Note the absence of the posterior part and splenium of the corpus callosum associated with medial radiating sulci (white open arrows). A large interhemispheric CSF-containing space communicates with an enlarged cistern velum interpositum. The massa intermedia is enlarged (white arrow). Note also the beaked tectum, barely visible aqueduct, a collapsed non-visible fourth ventricle, an inferior vermial peg (black open arrow) and a cervico-medullary kink (curved arrow).

should not be interpreted as periaqueductal CSF absorption (16). Direct observation of CSF movement can be inferred from the appearance of an absent signal within the aqueduct and third ventricle due to pulsatile and bidirectional CSF flow (Fig. 3.6D) (7). This sign was reported in the majority of patients with hydrocephalus but unfortunately was also seen in almost half the patients with cerebral atrophy and in some normal patients (7). Another and more reliable but invasive method for demonstrating the functional patency of the aqueduct is to inject a small amount of a dilute water-soluble contrast agent into the lateral ventricle and follow with CT scanning (Fig. 3.7). Opacification of the third but not of the fourth ventricle indicates occlusion of the aqueduct.

Dandy-Walker Malformation

The features of the Dandy-Walker malformation—absence of the inferior vermis; widely separated cerebellar nodules; cystic dilatation of the fourth ventricle; and hydrocephalus involving the lateral and third ventricles—are

easily determined by CT or MRI (Fig. 3.8). Elevation of the torcular, which is an important feature (as would be the presence of hydrocephalus) in differentiating the Dandy-Walker syndrome from primary cerebellar vermial agenesis, is easily defined by sagittal plane MRI.

Aneurysm of the Great Vein of Galen

An aneurysm of the great vein of Galen is considered by many to be the result of a arteriovenous malformation at the posterior margin of the tentorium in which an abnormal communication between the posterior choroidal branches of the posterior cerebral arteries and the great vein exists. As a result the vein becomes enormously enlarged and can compress the cerebral aqueduct and posterior third ventricle, with consequent hydrocephalus. On CT the aneurysm is diagnosed and an enhancing posterior third ventricular mass with enlargement of the lateral and third ventricles. On MRI the lesion is seen as a low-intensity lesion on both T1 and T2 scans—the low intensity representing a flow-void phenomenon due to rapid blood flow (Fig. 3.9).

Post-inflammatory/Hemorrhagic Obstruction

Following ventriculitis the ventricular system may be blocked at the foramen of Monro, the aqueduct, or at the exit foramina from the fourth ventricle (Fig. 3.7). The level of the obstruction can be determined with CT by noting ventricular enlargement proximal to the obstruction. On occasion both the aqueduct and the outlet foramina of the fourth ventricle may be blocked. The fourth ventricle is then trapped and develops a distinctive ovoid configuration (Fig. 3.10). The most common type of hemorrhage causing ventricular dilatation in the pediatric age group is that following neonatal germinal matrix hemorrhage with ventricular extension. Ultrasound is excellent to show the ventricles' size and the hemorrhage site (Fig. 3.11).

Tumors

Cerebral tumors causing hydrocephalus frequently occur in the posterior fossa. Both CT and MRI are excellent diagnostic tests, (Fig. 3.12), but MRI is probably the preferred of the two because its sagittal plane imaging can pre-

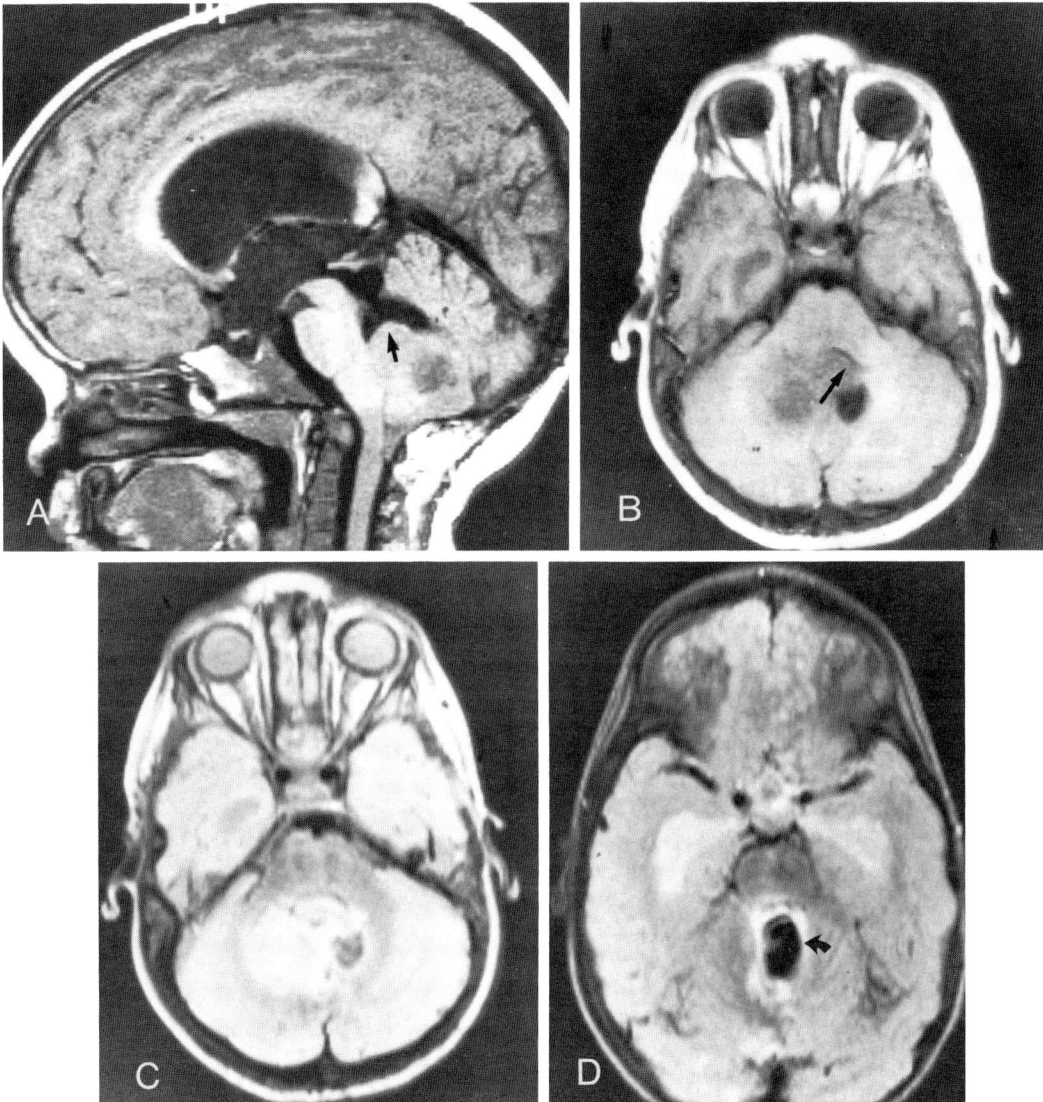

Figure 3.6.   *A*. Sagittal plane MR, T1-weighted scan, demonstrates a tumor with a low-intensity center displacing the fourth ventricle superiorly (arrow). Note the hydrocephalus and the dilatation of the aqueduct. *B*. An axial T1-weighted scan demonstrates the low intensity tumor displacing the fourth ventricle to the right (arrow). *C*. On a T2-weighted scan the tumor is seen as a high-intensity lesion. *D*. On a T2-weighted image 8 mm higher through the fourth ventricle, the signal loss (arrow) is probably due to excessive pulsatile flow above the obstruction.

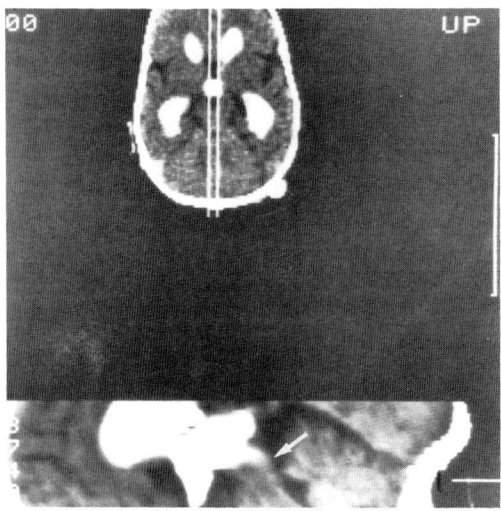

Figure 3.7. A contrast-enhanced CT ventriculogram shows an obstruction at the level of the aqueduct (arrow) in a 3-month-old child with aqueduct stenosis due to strepto-coccal meningitis.

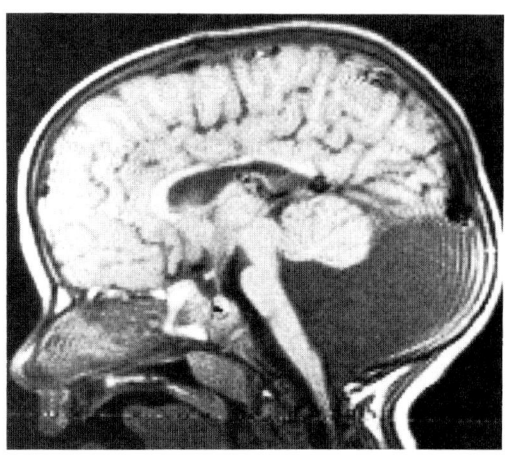

Figure 3.8. A sagittal plane MRI scan demonstrates absence of the inferior vermis with direct communication between a large cystic space and the fourth ventricle (arrows). Hydrocephalus is not evident on this midline image but was seen on parasagittal images.

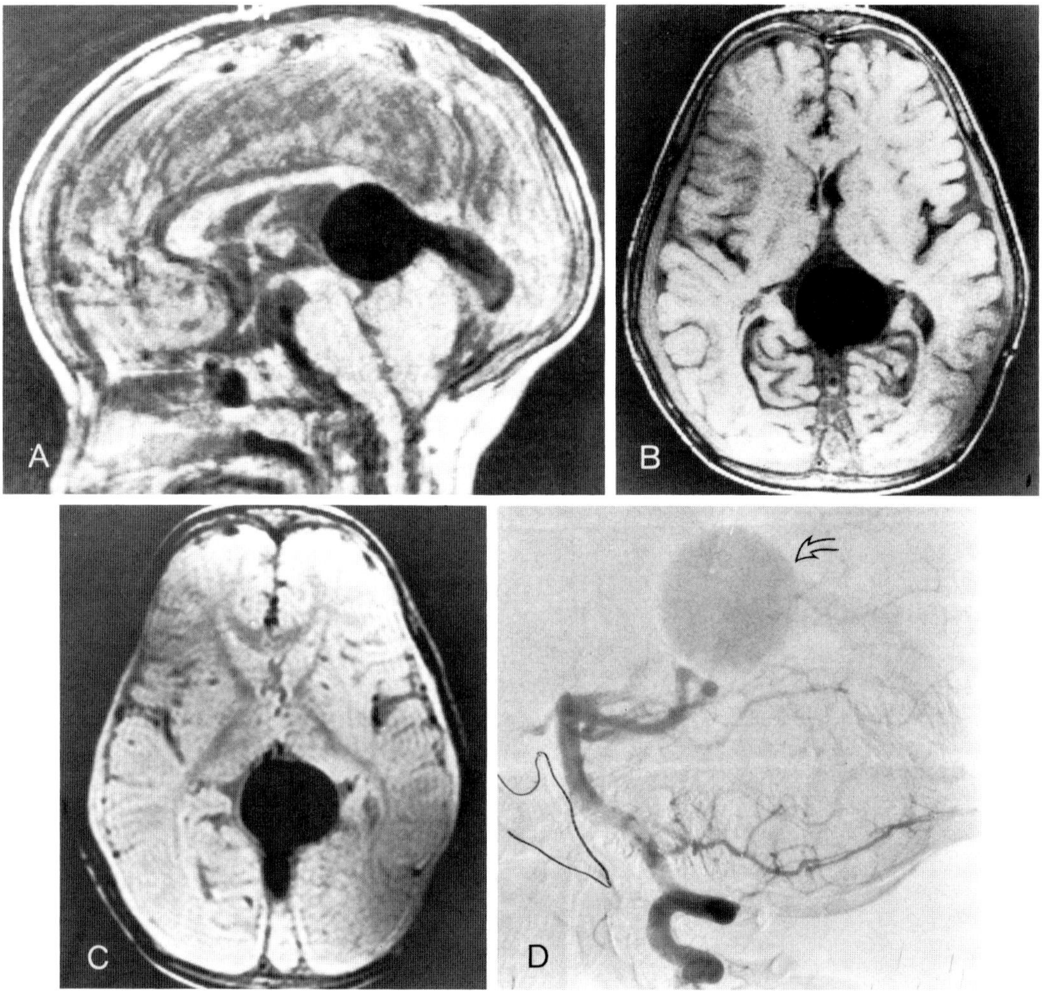

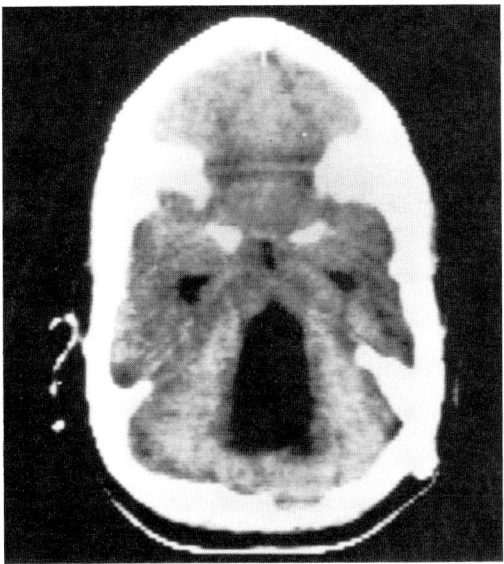

Figure 3.10.   Note the enlarged 4th ventricle due to obstruction of the aqueduct and of the outlet foramina of the ventricle in a child with Chiari II malformation. (A similar appearance would be found in a case of ventriculitis with aqueductal and foraminal blockage.)

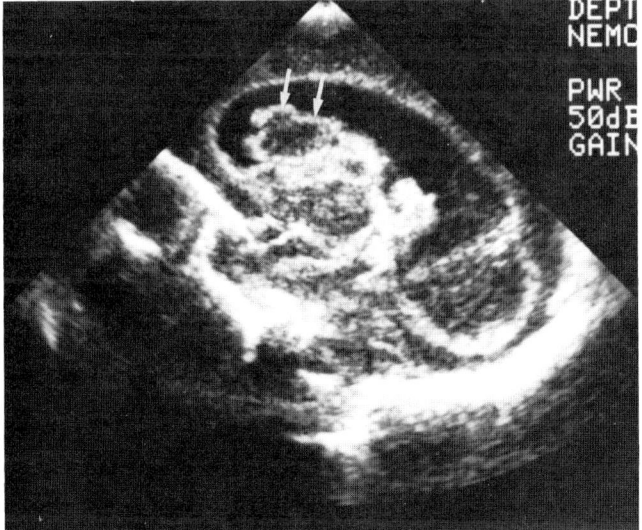

Figure 3.11. A sagittal plan ultrasound image demonstrates a cavitating hemorrhage (arrows) underlying an enlarged lateral ventricle. The cavitation is due to breakdown of the hemorrhage.

Figure 3.9.   *A.* Sagittal plane MRI, T1-weighted scan demonstrates a large aneurysm of the great Vein of Galen with some enlargement of the straight sinus as well. *B.* Axial T1-weighted and *C.* T2-weighted scans again demonstrate the aneurysm. The lack of signal in all three images represents rapidly flowing blood. *D.* Vertebral angiography confirmed the presence of the aneurysm (arrow).

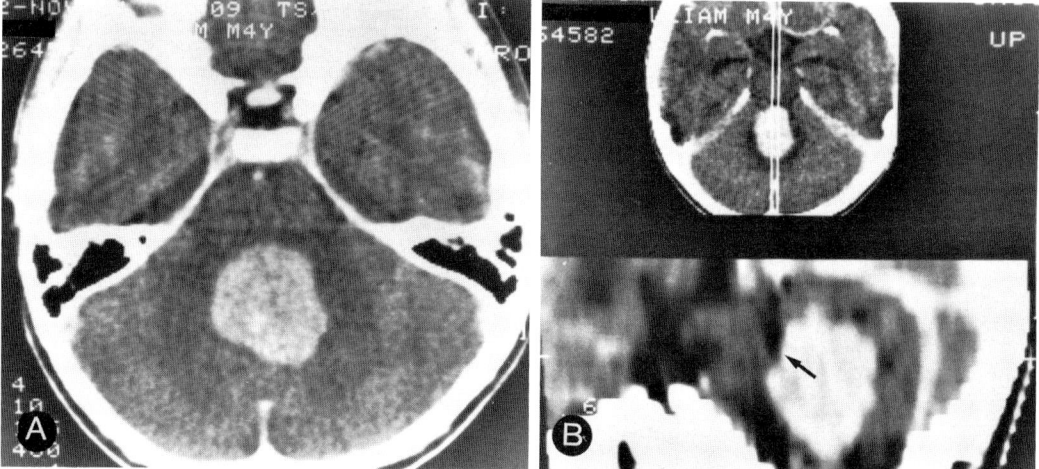

Figure 3.12. *A.* A contrast enhanced axial CT scan and *B.* a sagittal reformatted scan demonstrates a large contrast-enhancing tumor displacing the fourth ventricle (arrow) superiorly.

cisely show the extent of the tumor into the fourth ventricle, pons, or midbrain (Fig. 3.6). However, the calcification often seen with certain tumors (such as ependymomas) cannot be determined reliably with MRI scanning. The contrast enhancement seen on CT after the injection of an intravenous iodinated contrast medium in patients with medulloblastomas, ependymomas, and astrocytomas can now be matched with MRI scans using the agent Gadolinium-DTPA.

Hydrocephalus can also follow obstructions at the level of the third ventricle, as seen with pineal region tumors, or at the level of the aqueduct (periaqueductal glioma). Both CT and MRI can define these lesions accurately, again with MRI having the added benefit of sagittal plane imaging.

EXTERNAL OBSTRUCTIVE (COMMUNICATING) HYDROCEPHALUS

Congenital Anomalies

Arachnoid cysts in or near the CSF pathways may obstruct them with resultant hydrocephalus (Fig. 3.13). Specifically, hydrocephalus is often seen with arachnoid cysts behind the cerebellum and with cysts involving the suprasellar cisterns. Retrocerebellar cysts (Fig. 3.14) are considered by some to represent persistence of Blake's pouch—an embryologically-derived structure that represents evagination of the roof of the fourth ventricle extending upward and posterior into the primitive meninx caudal to the cerebellum (4). The pouch usually communicates with the sub-

arachnoid space between the eighth and sixteenth gestational week. If the ventricular orifice of this cystic structure remains small or becomes separated from the roof of the fourth ventricle, CSF secretion from the choroid plexus contained within the cyst may enlarge it. If the cyst wall tears, communication with the subarachnoid space occurs. Since the tentorium adheres to the inner table of the skull at its adult position at the end of the first trimester, the torcular is often elevated. CT diagnosis of an arachnoid cyst is easy, particularly if sagittal reformatted images are available. If the tentorium is not elevated, the retrocerebellar CSF collection is most likely due to an enlarged cisterna magna.

Suprasellar arachnoid cysts are probably secondary to adhesive arachnoiditis at the level of the chiasmatic cistern. As a result, the suprasellar and interpeduncular cisterns dilate to form a cystic structure easily seen on CT or MRI (Fig. 3.3). Indentation of the third ventricle by the cyst accounts for the accompanying hydrocephalus.

Post-inflammatory Hydrocephalus

A basal meningitis usually due to infection with *Escherichia coli, Staphylococus aureus, Streptococcus pneumococcus,* or *Haemophilus influenza* (21) will cause a communicating external hydrocephalus if the basal cisterns are occluded. Radiologically mild-to-moderate ventriculomegaly with enlargement of the basal cisterns, the subarachnoid space in the frontal and frontoparietal regions, and the interhemispheric fissure frontally is seen (Fig. 3.15). The communicating hydrocephalus may resolve, progress, or evolve to a picture of cerebral atrophy.

The size of the subarachnoid spaces in children is variable and radiological findings similar to communicating hydrocephalus are occasionally seen in normal patients (15). In questionable cases, examination of the occipitofrontal head circumference, and particularly its relation to standard growth curves, should help distinguish the pathological from the normal. The differentiation of communicating hy-

drocephalus from cerebral atrophy in the pediatric age group is helped by noting that the extracerebral subarachnoid spaces are wide throughout the hemispheres in patients with atrophy (Fig. 3.16), whereas in the benign "external hydrocephalus," the widening is mainly frontal and the *anterior* interhemispheric fissure is wide (Fig. 3.15) (18). In most patients with communicating hydrocephalus the fourth ventricle is not enlarged (23). A practical and frequent dilemma is to distinguish benign external hydrocephalus from chronic subdural hygromas. The CT appearances may be identi-

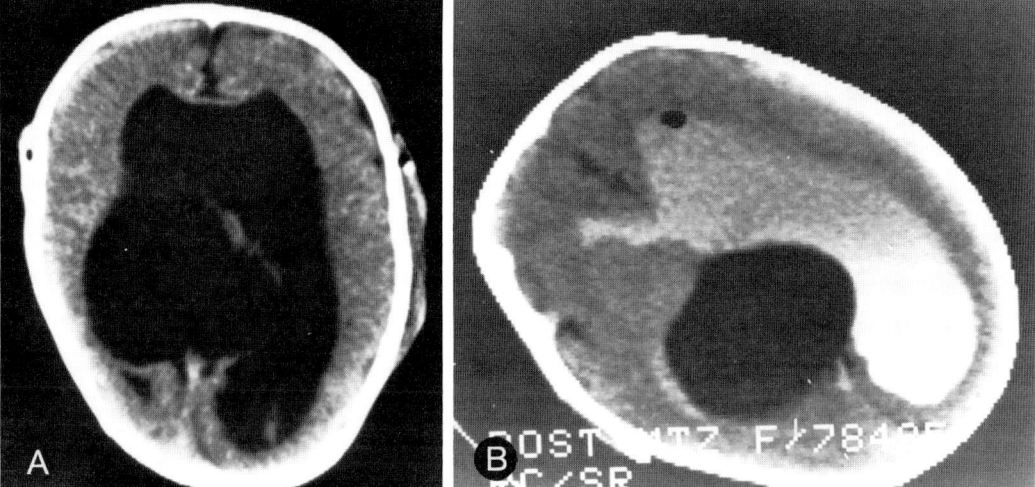

Figure 3.13. *A.* Marked hydrocephalus and an extraventricular fluid-containing cavity is seen on an axial CT scan. *B.* After metrizamide was injected into the lateral ventricles an arachnoid cyst probably derived from the ambient cistern is identified.

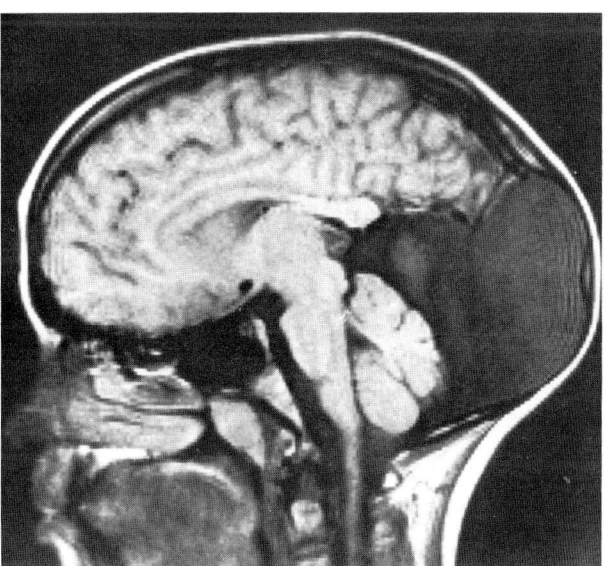

Figure 3.14. A sagittal plane MRI scan demonstrates a large retrocerebellar cyst displacing the cerebellum anteriorly. Mild hydrocephalus was seen on the axial scans.

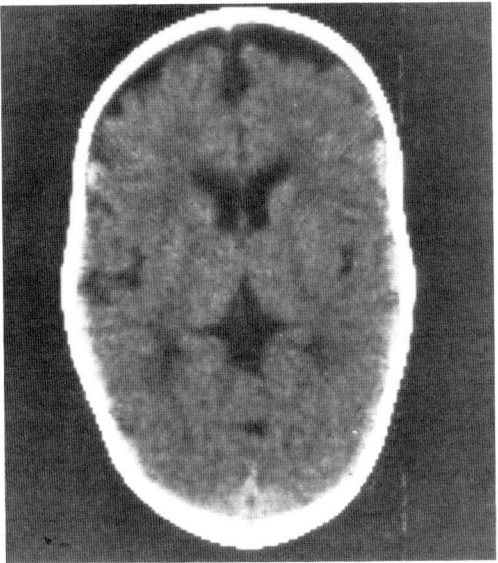

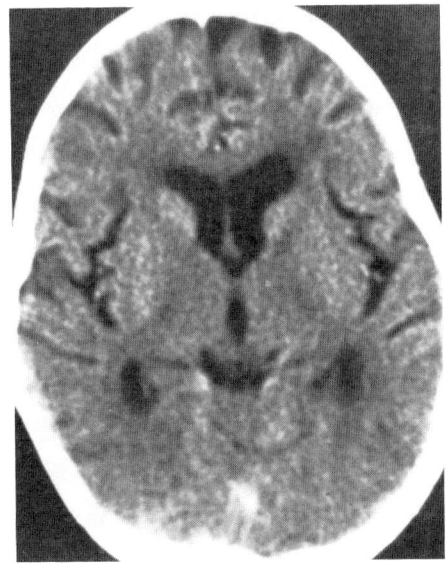

Figure 3.15. A non-enhanced axial CT scan demonstrates mild ventriculomegaly and widening of the frontal and anterior interhemispheric subarachnoid spaces in a 1-year-old child with H. flu meningitis.

Figure 3.16. Note the generalized widening of the sulci with moderate ventriculomegaly due to cerebral atrophy in a 12-year-old female who underwent radiation therapy for acute lymphocytic leukemia.

cal or the two conditions may coexist, and the diagnosis must be made on clinical grounds. In a number of children with macrocephaly, CT demonstrates changes identical to that of post-inflammatory communicating hydrocephalus—i.e., enlargement of the subarachnoid spaces with mild ventriculomegaly. However, there is no history of meningitis and the course is usually benign. In a significant number of these infants there is a familiar occurrence of enlarged heads (2, 18). Evidence of elevated ICP is minimal.

Post-hemorrhagic Obstruction

Blood in the basal cisterns alone is considered to be a rare cause of infantile hydrocephalus (17). Probably head trauma is the most common cause for subarachnoid blood in the pediatric and adult age group, and hydrocephalus may follow the accompanying arachnoid inflammatory reaction. Frequently, the hydrocephalus seen following trauma is due to a hydrocephalus ex-vacuo following brain injury, gliosis, and tissue loss.

Venous Thrombosis

There is considerable controversy as to whether elevated venous pressure secondary to venous thrombosis can cause hydrocephalus.

Experimentally Bering and Salibi (3) produced ventricular enlargement in dogs by occluding both jugular veins. Acute sinus thrombosis, on the other hand, produces primarily cerebral edema and not hydrocephalus (14). Rosman and Shands showed that the patient's age is critical in determining whether cerebral venous hypertension causes hydrocephalus (in infants under 18 months) or pseudotumor cerebri (in older children) (32). Sinus thrombosis in patients with hydrocephalus can be diagnosed by the failure of sinus opacification on contrast-enhanced CT, by the demonstration of an increased signal intensity in the sinus on both T1 and T2-weighted MRI scans, or by the absence of opacification of the sinuses on cerebral angiography. A contiguous cortical vein thrombosis can be suggested when a low-density area is seen by CT at the gray-white junction indicating an associated cortical infarct.

Tumors

Patients with carcinomatous meningitis from neoplastic involvement of the basal cisterns may develop a communicating hydrocephalus. CT with contrast enhancement will demonstrate focal or generalized enhancement of basal cisterns or cortical subarachnoid spaces.

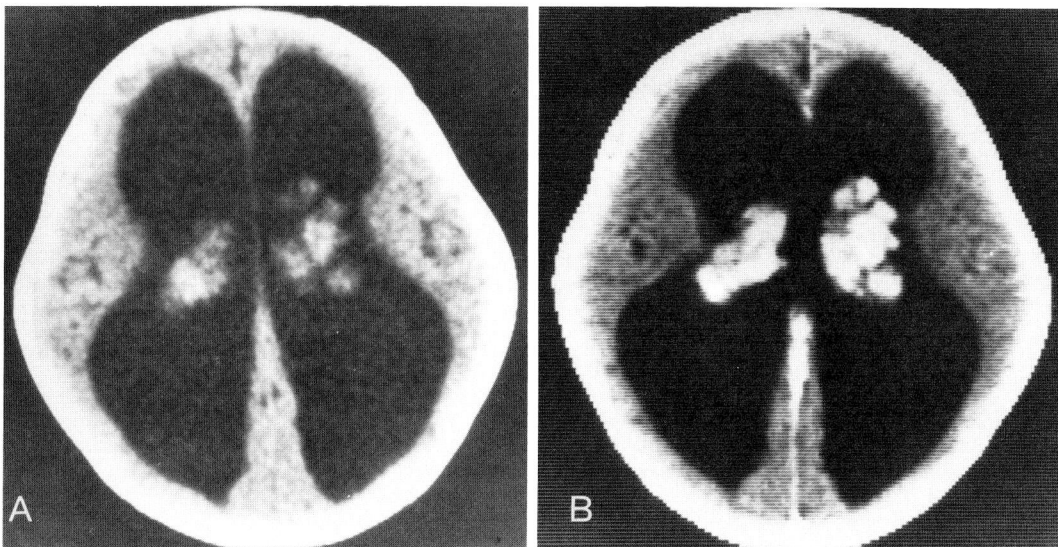

Figure 3.17. *A.* On a non-enhanced CT scan, massive enlargement of the ventricles is seen. Note also the bilaterally enlarged choroid plexus containing calcification. *B.* With contrast medium the choroid plexus is enhanced. At surgery choroid plexus papillomas were resected.

NON-OBSTRUCTIVE (ATROPHIC) HYDROCEPHALUS

Also known as hydrocephalus ex-vacuo, this form is due to loss of brain tissue. Most of these cases are caused by vascular insufficiency and are evaluated equally well by CT and MRI.

Functional Hydrocephalus

Excessive secretion of CSF by a tumor such as a choroid plexus papilloma is the sine qua non of functional hydrocephalus. The condition can be diagnosed by CT when a densely enhancing, enlarged choroid plexus is seen in association with enlargement of the lateral ventricles. Large tumor masses in the lateral ventricles may also be seen on MRI (Fig. 3.17).

Impaired absorption of CSF may be due to congenital aplasia of the arachnoid villi (10). The results of such a deficiency will be evident on CT as a communicating hydrocephalus.

REFERENCES

1. Asada, M., Tamaki, N., Kanazawa, Y., *et al.* Computer analysis of periventricular lucency on the CT scan. Neuroradiology, *16*:207–211, 1978.
2. Barlow, C.F. CSF Dynamics in hydrocephalus with special attention to external hydrocephalus. Brain Dev., *6*:119–127, 1984.
3. Bering, E.A.J. and Salibi, B. Production of hydrocephalus by increased cephalic-venous pressure. Arch. Neurol. Psychiat., *81*:693–698, 1959.
4. Coben, L.A. Absence of a foramen of Magendie in the dog, cat, rabbit, and goat. Arch. Neurol., *16*:524–528, 1967.
5. Di Rocco, C., Di Trapani, G., Pettorossi, V.E., *et al.* On the pathology of experimental hydrocephalus induced by artificial increase in endoventricular CSF pulse pressure. Child's Brain, *5*:81–95, 1979.
6. Draver, B.P., Rosenbaum, A.E., Reigel, D.B., *et al.* Metrizamide computed tomography cisternography: pediatric applications. Radiology, *124*:349–357, 1977.
7. El Gammal, T., Allen, M.B., Brooks, B.S., *et al.* MR evaluation of hydrocephalus. Am. J. Neurorad., *8*:591–597, 1987.
8. Emery, J.L. Intracranial effects of long-standing decompression of the brain in children with hydrocephalus and menigomyelocele. Dev. Med. Child Neurol., *7*:302–309, 1965.
9. Fitz, C.R., Harwood-Nash, D.C., Chuang, S., *et al.* Metrizamide ventriculography and computed tomography in infants and children. Neuroradiology, *16*:6–9, 1978.
10. Gilles, F.H. and Davidson, R.I. Communicating hydrocephalus associated with deficient dysplastic parasagittal arachnoidal granulations. J. Neurosurg., *35*:421–426, 1971.
11. Gilles, F.H. and Gilles, E.E. Hydrocephalus in the neonate, infant and child. In *Disorders of the Developing Nervous System: Diagnosis and Treatment,* edited by H.J. Hoffman and F. Epstein, p. 541. Blackwell Scientific Publications, Boston, 1986.
12. Hiratuska, H.J., Fujiwara, K., and Okada, K. Modification of periventricular hypodensity in hydrocephalus with ventricular reflux in metrizamide CT cisternography. J. Comput. Assist. Tomogr., *3*:204–208, 1979.
13. Hiratuski, H.J., Tabata, H., Tsuruoka, S., Aoyagi, M., *et al.* Evaluation of periventricular hypodensity in experimental hydrocephalus by metrizamide CT

ventriculography. J. Neurosurg., *56*:235–240, 1982.

14. Kalbag, F.M. and Woolf, A.L. Primary thrombosis of the dural sinuses in adult life. In: *Cerebral Venous Thrombosis*, edited by R.M. Kalbag and A.L. Woolf, p. 46. London, Oxford University Press, 1967.

15. Kingsley, D. and Kendall, B.E. The value of computed tomography in the evaluation of the enlarged head. Neuroradiology, *15*:59–71, 1978.

16. Lee, B.C.P. Magnetic resonance imaging of periaqueductal lesions. Clin. Radiol., *38*:527–533, 1987.

17. Lorber, J. and Bassi, U. The aetiology of neonatal hydrocephalus (excluding cases of spina bifida). Dev. Med. Child Neurol., *7*:289–294, 1965.

18. Maytal, J., Alvarez, L.A., Elkin, C.M., *et al*. External hydrocephalus: radiologic spectrumand differentiation from cerebral atrophy. Amer. J. Roentgenol., *148*:1223–1230, 1987.

19. McClone, D.G., Bondareff, W., and Raimondi, A.J. Hydrocephalus-3, a murine mutant: II. Changes in the brain extracellular space. Surg. Neurol., *1*:233–242, 1973.

20. McComb, J.G. Physiology of cerebrospinal fluid circulation. In: Hoffman, H.J., Epstein, E. (eds): *Disorders of the Developing Nervous System: Diagnosis and Treatment*, edited by H.J. Hoffman and E. Epstein, p. 483. Boston, Blackwell Scientific Publications, 1986.

21. Milhorat, T.H. Pathology of hydrocephalus. In: *Hydrocephalus and the Cerebrospinal Fluid*. edited by T.H. Milhorat, p.63. Baltimore, Williams & Wilkins, 1972.

22. Mori, K., Murata, T., and Nakano, Y. Periventricular lucency in computed tomography of hydrocephalus and cerebral atrophy. J. Comput. Assist. Tomogr., *4*:204–209, 1980.

23. Naidich, T.P., Schott, L.H., and Baron, R.L. Computed tomography in evaluation of hydrocephalus. Radio. Clin. North Am., *20*:143–167, 1982.

24. Naidich, T.P., Epstein, F., and Lin, J.P. Evaluation of pediatric hydrocephalus by computed tomography. Radiology, *119*:337–345, 1976.

25. Naidich, T.P., McClone, D.G., Hahn, Y.S., *et al*. Atrial diverticula in severe hydrocephalus. Amer. J. Neurorad., *3*:257–266, 1982.

26. Naidich, T.P. and McLone, D.G. Radiographic classification and gross morphologic features of hydrocephalus. In: *Disorders of the Developing Nervous System: Diagnosis and Treatment* edited by H.J. Hoffman and F. Epstein, p. 505. Boston, Blackwell Scientific Publications, 1986.

27. Oi, S. and Matsumoto, S. Morphological findings of postshunt slit-like ventricle in experimental canine hydrocephalus. Child's Nerv. Syst., *2*:179–184, 1986.

28. Pedersen, H., Gyldenstedt, M., and Gyldenstedt, C. Measurement of the normal ventricular system and supratentorial subarachnoid space in children with computed tomography. Neuroradiology., *17*:231–237, 1979.

29. Penn, R.D. and Bacus, J.W. The brain as a sponge: a computed tomographic look at Hakin's hypothesis. Neurosurgery., *14*:670–674, 1984.

30. Reulen, H.J., Tsuyunu, M., Tack, A., et al. Clearance of edema fluid into cerebrospinal fluid. A mechanism for the resolution of vasogenic brain edema. J. Neurosurg., *48*:754–764, 1978.

31. Rosenberg, G.A., Kyner, W.T., and Estrada, E. Bulk flow of brain interstitial fluid under normal and hyperosmolar conditions. Am. J. Physiol., *238*:F42–F49, 1980.

32. Rosman, N.P. and Shands K.N. Hydrocephalus caused by increased intracranial venous pressure: a clinico-pathologic study. Ann. Neurol., *3*:445–450, 1978.

33. Russell, D.S. *Observations on the Pathology of Hydrocephalus*. Her Majesty's Stationery Office (Special Report Series Medical Research Council, no. 265), London, 1949.

34. Smith, J.R.L., Haber, K., Reynolds, A.F., *et al*. Ultrasonic evaluation of postventricular shunt dynamics in infants and young children. Radiology, *145*:133–138, 1982.

35. Takei, F., Shapiro, K., and Kohn, I. Influence of the rate of ventricular enlargement on the white matter water content in progressive feline hydrocephalus. J. Neurosurg., *66*:577–583, 1987.

36. Takei, F., Shapiro, K., Hirano, A., *et al*. Influence of the rate of ventricular enlargement on the ultrastructural morphology of the white matter in experimental hydrocephalus. Neurosurgery, *21*:645–650, 1987.

37. Weller, R.O. and Shulman, K. Infantile hydrocephalus: clinical, histological, and ultrastructural study of brain damage. J. Neurosurg., *36*:255–265, 1972.

CHAPTER 4

Medical Treatment of Hydrocephalus

HERBERT E. GILMORE, M.D.

INTRODUCTION

The role of medical therapy for the treatment of hydrocephalus remains uncertain despite its use for over 30 years. There have been no studies comparing short- or long-term outcomes of surgical and medical treatments, but the natural course of untreated hydrocephalus is well documented (15, 37, 75). Approximately 50% of untreated patients die as a direct result of hydrocephalus and the remaining 50% survive with "arrested hydrocephalus." Of the latter, only 11%-18% have normal cognitive and neurologic findings when examined at follow-up (15, 73). The remaining 82%-89% have varying degrees of cognitive delay and neurological abnormalities, which may not become apparent until years after the presumed "arrest" of hydrocephalus (29). The adverse effects of hydrocephalus on cerebral white matter (and to a lesser extent, on gray matter) have been well documented (17, 28, 32, 44, 49, 51, 52, 55, 59, 64, 66, 68, 70, 71, 72), and include ultrastructural and biochemical changes that may be irreversible if hydrocephalus is untreated. Therefore investigators agree that most patients with hydrocephalus require either surgical or medical treatment. Indeed, some investigators argue for early treatment of all hydrocephalus to prevent such changes (22, 51, 55, 58, 59, 71, 76). There is no consensus, however, as to which treatment is better or in which circumstance one or the other should be used.

One major obstacle in comparing various studies is a lack of uniform definition of hydrocephalus. Some investigators limit the definition to include only cases in which symptoms and signs of increased intracranial pressure (ICP) are present, while others have included all cases in which ventricular dilatation is present with or without clinical symptoms of increased ICP. Indeed, most investigators do not define ventricular dilatation, nor do they indicate how estimations of ventricular size are ascertained. Additionally, most studies do not define hydrocephalus using ICP measurements.

Patients with rapidly progressive hydrocephalus and symptoms of increased ICP require either ventricular drainage or shunt surgery (2, 35). Some patients, particularly infants, with transient hydrocephalus following intraventricular hemorrhage (IVH) may never require any form of treatment (1). Others with slowly progressive hydrocephalus may not require immediate treatment. There are no criteria with which to predict who will have transient or slowly progressive hydrocephalus and who will have a more rapid course. In addition, no guidelines have been established to determine the type of medical treatment related to the type of hydrocephalus, the timing and the duration of treatment, the outcome variables to be followed, or the duration of follow-up.

The goal in treating hydrocephalus medically is to reduce ventricular size and decrease ICP so that acceptable neurological and cognitive outcomes result with fewer side effects than those that sometimes follow shunt surgery. Sequelae of shunt surgery can be significant and include frequent shunt revision, meningitis, and ventriculitis (4, 19, 24, 27, 30, 31). In the first 6-12 months of life the treatment goal is to halt the progression of hydrocephalus until it arrests spontaneously. The potential for spontaneous arrest of hydrocephalus exists in infants, since there is a linear increase in absorption of cerebrospinal fluid (CSF) with increasing ICP (14, p.37). As the sutures become fibrotic with age, ICP increases to adult levels and CSF absorption likewise increases. Thus, a new equilibrium is established between CSF production and absorption at a ventricular volume and an ICP that is not deleterious to the brain, obviating the need for shunt surgery. In older patients the therapeutic goal is less clear, since the ultimate equilibrium between production and absorption of CSF has already been established.

Lacking comparative studies, a discussion of the medical management of hydrocephalus comparing various medical treatments to each other and to shunt surgery is not possible. The most that can be achieved is a presentation of the effects and side-effects of various treatments and of the outcome of patients so treated, when such data are available.

The four principal categories of medical treatment of hydrocephalus are based on *a*) removal of CSF, *b*) decrease in CSF production, *c*) decrease in cerebral water content, and *d*) increase in CSF absorption.

TREATMENT TO REMOVE CSF

CSF is formed mainly in the choroid plexus of the cerebral ventricular system and to a lesser extent at extra-choroidal sites, at a rate of 0.02 ml/min in neonates and 0.35 ml/min in adults (14). CSF absorption occurs mainly at the arachnoid villi and partly through the brain interstitial spaces via transependymal flow at a rate equal to the rate of production. The total amount of CSF present in the ventricles varies from 5-15 ml in neonates to 150 ml in adults.

Non-surgical removal of CSF by serial lumbar puncture (LP) has been advocated for the treatment of hydrocephalus secondary to IVH in infants and for the treatment of normal pressure hydrocephalus (NPH) in adults. In the former, hydrocephalus is caused by blockage of CSF absorption due to fibrin deposition at the arachnoid villi. The rationale for repeated LPs is to decrease protein and blood in the CSF and thereby prevent the formation of fibrin (16, 46). In NPH, the mechanism of hydrocephalus is unknown but is presumed to also be blockage of CSF absorption at the arachnoid villi (20). The amount of CSF recommended for removal with each LP varies from 1-15 ml in neonates with post-hemorrhagic hydrocephalus (PHH) to 40-50 ml in adults with NPH.

Serial Lumbar Puncture

Mantovani et al, in an attempt to *prevent* the development of PHH in 19 infants, initiated daily LPs within 24 hours of demonstrating IVH by computerized tomography (CT) (46). Only infants with at least grade II IVH (blood filling 10%-50% of the lateral ventricle) were included in the study. Three to 5 ml of CSF were removed over several minutes until the CSF was clear and had a protein content less than 180 mg/dl. An equal number of infants with comparable degree of IVH were given supportive treatment only without serial LP. No differences in mortality or frequency of hydrocephalus were noted between the treated and untreated groups. Only 7 of 38 infants (18%) who developed hydrocephalus required shunt surgery. The results of this study were complicated by the fact that glycerol was given after LPs were discontinued. Similar results were obtained in another study of 47 infants with at least grade III IVH (ventricular hemorrhage and dilation) (3). In 24 of these infants CSF was removed by LP until flow ceased (1-5 ml). The LPs were performed every other day until ventricular size decreased, as measured by cerebral ultrasound or until clinical signs of increased ICP developed, necessitating shunt surgery. In 23 of the infants supportive care only was given. Eleven of the 47 patients (4 control and 7 treated) developed hydrocephalus (23%). Six of the 11 patients (3 control and 3 treated) required shunt surgery. In neither study were data presented regarding the long-term follow up of these infants. Therefore, no statement can be made regarding the effect of serial LPs on developmental and neurological outcomes of infants with PHH, though both studies clearly demonstrate the ineffectiveness of such therapy in *preventing* PHH.

Once PHH has *developed* in premature infants following IVH, LPs can temporarily reduce ventricular dilation and alleviate symptoms of increased ICP until spontaneous resolution of hydrocephalus occurs or until shunt surgery can be performed. In one study the effectiveness of treating *transient* PHH by single, widely-spaced LPs in 3 infants was demonstrated (16). Five to 15 ml of CSF were removed with each LP. In another study 11 of 15 infants with PHH had an arrest in progression of hydrocephalus as demonstrated by CT following serial LPs (53). Daily LPs were performed beginning at a mean of 15 days of age and continuing for a mean of 23 days. The amount of CSF removed was 30-98 ml/week. Only 1 treated and 3 untreated infants required shunt surgery. Kreusser et al demonstrated that after PHH had developed, removal of large amounts of CSF (15 ml/kg) by daily LPs resulted in either reduction in, or stabilization of, ventricular size until shunt surgery could be performed more safely (36). Using serial cranial ultrasound, they demonstrated that a reduction in ventricular size following an LP could predict stabilization of ventricular size. All 4 patients in whom such a reduction in ventricular size following LP could *not* be demonstrated, required either shunt surgery (3 patients) or ventricular drainage (1 patient). There was no control group of patients in this study.

It is difficult to compare the results of these studies since the grading of IVH, the definition of hydrocephalus, the amount of CSF removed, the duration of treatment, and the duration and type of follow-up vary widely. Nonetheless, they do suggest that serial LPs may be efficacious for the temporary control of PHH once hydrocephalus has been demonstrated, as long as relatively large amounts of CSF are removed and as long as cranial ultrasound can demonstrate a reduction in ventricular size following such removal. However, the duration of the benefit is uncertain, while side effects of serial LPs have been documented. In one study meningitis was identified in 6 of 22 infants (27%) who had undergone a mean of 16 LPs each (63). In another report vertebral osteomyelitis following 8 LPs for PHH was noted in one patient (6). MacMahon and Cooke reported significant hypernatremia as a complication of serial LPs in 3 infants. (43).

There are only a few reports of temporary relief of symptoms of NPH in adults using single or serial LPs. All patients ultimately came to shunt surgery with variable improvement in their symptoms. In one study removal of 40-50 ml CSF and a battery of psychometric tests were used to predict the success of later shunt surgery in patients with NPH (74). There are no studies in which LPs alone have been used as a permanent treatment for NPH.

TREATMENT TO DECREASE CSF PRODUCTION

About two thirds of CSF is formed at the choroid plexus and the other third is formed in the brain and spinal cord (14). Choroidal production involves three processes: *a*) filtration of water across the choroidal capillary cell wall, influenced principally by hydrostatic pressure, *b*) active transport of water and ions across the choroidal epithelium, controlled mainly by Na^+/K^+ ATPase, and *c*) active secretion of water and ions by the choroidal epithelium into the ventricles, controlled chiefly by the activity of carbonic anhydrase. Although there are no reported therapeutic benefits of altering the first process, reductions in the latter processes have been achieved experimentally and clinically to decrease CSF production significantly. Of the two processes, inhibition of carbonic anhydrase activity has been more extensively studied and used than inhibition of Na^+/K^+ ATPase.

Carbonic Anhydrase Inhibitors

Various inhibitors of carbonic anhydrase activity have been described and studied in great detail (47). Only two of these substances, acetazolamide and furosemide, have been used therapeutically to reduce CSF production. Acetazolamide is a more potent carbonic anhydrase inhibitor than furosemide by 10 to 100-fold (47). Yet, furosemide is as potent an inhibitor of CSF formation, suggesting that it may inhibit CSF production and secretion at another, as yet undetermined, step in the pathway of CSF formation (57). Both drugs can reduce CSF flow by 50%-60% at doses sufficient to decrease carbonic anhydrase activity by 98% with furosemide and 99.5% with acetazolamide (45). Preferential vasoconstriction of the choroidal arteries is another effect of acetazolamide that may further reduce CSF production. Various dosage regimens have been recommended for both drugs to achieve such inhibition: 50-150 mg/kg for acetazolamide and 1 mg/kg for furosemide. The onset of reduction in CSF flow is within 30-40 minutes after either drug is given intravenously; the maximum effect occurs within 70-90 minutes (45). The duration of action of both drugs ranges from 30 minutes to greater than 2.5 hours. Both drugs affect processes throughout the body so that significant metabolic side effects can potentially occur with their use. Acetazolamide can cause metabolic acidosis by increasing bicarbonate loss through the kidney and increasing hydrogen ion in the blood. Volpe has expressed concern that high-dose acetazolamide treatment may have a potential toxic effect on myelin in infants (69). Furosemide can cause metabolic alkalosis by increasing hydrogen ion secretion in the kidney; it can also lead to nephrocalcinosis due to increased calcium excretion in the renal tubules (25).

Acetazolamide

Acetazolamide has been used as a diuretic since the 1950's. Tschirgi and associates first demonstrated its ability to significantly reduce CSF flow in cats and rabbits (67). Elvidge et al. reported its successful use in arresting hydrocephalus in a 4-year-old patient (11). Huttenlocher reported arrest in progression of hydrocephalus in 8 of 15 patients (53%) with *slowly* progressive hydrocephalus treated for as briefly as 6 months to as long as 2.5 years with an acetazolamide dose of 40-100 mg/kg/day (26). Some improvement in the progression of hydrocephalus was demonstrated in 2 of 15 patients (13%) and no improvement was noted in 5 patients (33%). He related the degree of improvement to the rate of head growth before treatment rather than to the dosage of acetazolamide, the timing of treatment, the duration of treatment, or the type of hydrocephalus treated. Those patients with head growth greater than 1.5 cm/month failed treatment, whereas those with a growth rate of 1-1.5 cm/month had borderline improvement and those with a rate less than 1 cm/month had complete control of hydrocephalus. He noted tachypnea and metabolic acidosis in all patients receiving at least 50 mg/kg/day. All patients with *rapid* head growth had shunt surgery performed initially. Likewise, Mealey and Barker demonstrated that acetazolamide was ineffective in preventing the progression of hydrocephalus in 15 patients with myelomeningocele, who had *rapidly* progressive head growth (greater than 5 cm/month), and who were treated within the first week of life (48).

In these studies, the terms *slowly* and *rapidly* progressive hydrocephalus were never defined. Although several of the patients studied demonstrated improvement in neurological and cognitive abilities, outcomes were not followed systematically or prospectively. Also, no attempt was made to compare the outcome of surgical treatment of rapidly progressive hydrocephalus to acetazolamide treatment of slowly progressive hydrocephalus. Additionally, there was inconsistent documentation of decrease in ventricular size in patients with an arrest in progression of head growth. One must assume that the arrest in head growth was due to decrease in ventricular size but this was not looked for consistently. Donat did report such a decrease in ventricular size by CT before and after treatment with 100 mg/kg/day of acetazolamide (10). Although acidosis and mild dehydration developed in some of the patients studied, these side effects were not significant enough to warrant discontinuation of medication.

Acetazolamide and Furosemide

Shinnar et al reported a 51% success rate in avoiding shunt surgery in 49 patients with various types of hydrocephalus treated with acetazolamide (100 mg/kg/day) *and* furosemide (1 mg/kg/day) (60). The success rate in patients with hydrocephalus and myelomeningocele was only 26%. No patients with "transient hydrocephalus" were included; only patients who would have otherwise fulfilled the authors' criteria for shunt surgery were medically treated. Such therapy failed in all patients with *rapidly* progressive hydrocephalus. Metabolic acidosis, tachypnea and diarrhea were common, but were not severe enough to warrant discontinuation of therapy. The neurological and developmental outcomes of the medically treated and shunted patients in this study are unclear. The authors recommend medical therapy with these two agents for hydrocephalus *a)* in premature infants following IVH, since such infants may not tolerate shunt surgery, *b)* in all infants following meningitis, and *c)* in all infants with *slowly* progressive hydrocephalus. Although they did not study patients with transient hydrocephalus, they also recommend medical therapy for this condition following IVH. No mention was made of any infants developing nephrocalcinosis since they did not look specifically for this condition. Nephrocalcinosis has been reported in asphyxiated infants receiving 1.5-2 mg/kg/day furosemide for treatment of respiratory distress syndrome (25). In an ongoing, prospective study of early medical treatment of PHH, nephrocalcinosis has occurred frequently in pre-term infants treated with 1 mg/kg/day furosemide and 100 mg/kg/day acetazolamide (H. Gilmore, unpublished data). The long-term effect of nephrocalcinosis on renal function is unknown, as is the duration of furosemide-induced nephrocalcinosis.

Na^+/K^+ ATPase Inhibitors

Cardiac glycosides are the only Na^+/K^+ ATPase inhibitors that have been used for medical treatment of hydrocephalus. These drugs decrease CSF production by blocking the Na^+/K^+ ATPase transport of water and ions across the choroidal epithelium (14). The only drugs of this class that have been investigated are digoxin and ouabain. Most data regarding these drugs have come from animal experiments; only a few patients with hydrocephalus have been treated with them.

Digoxin and Ouabain

Neblett et al first noted that patients treated by ventricular drainage for hydrocephalus had a marked decrease in CSF flow when given digoxin (50). Similarly, topical application of ouabain to the choroid plexus in animals results in a significant reduction in CSF production (73). However, Bass et al reported the failure of 0.010-0.015 mg/kg/day digoxin to improve obstructive hydrocephalus in three infants (5). They investigated rapid head growth and symptoms of increased ICP. No studies were performed to assess decrease in ventricular size during treatment. No mention was made regarding the rate of progression of hydrocephalus or the duration of treatment. These same authors, however, reported a *profound* reduction in CSF production in rats given digoxin (5). Fifteen minutes after intravenous injection, the rate of CSF production fell by 50%; complete arrest of production was noted by 20-45 minutes; rapid recovery to resting levels occurred within 60 minutes. This effect on CSF production was not attributable to cardiotoxicity, since none was noted in any of the animals.

Despite this apparent dramatic effect on CSF production, no further studies have been performed using digoxin treatment in patients or experimental animals with hydrocephalus.

TREATMENT TO DECREASE BRAIN WATER CONTENT

Water is distributed in three compartments within the brain: a) the intracellular space, b) the interstitial space, and c) the cerebral blood vessels, mainly capillaries (14 pp. 113–131). The mechanisms that control the compartmentalization and flow of brain water have not been fully elucidated, but the osmotic gradient between each compartment plays a significant role. Obstruction of normal CSF flow in hydrocephalus results in transependymal flow of water and electrolytes from the ventricles into the interstitial space of the brain adjacent to the ventricular wall (14 pp. 113–131). Indeed, the CSF and the interstitial space are best considered a functional unit because of this free flow of water across the ependyma.

Osmotic diuretics may simply increase the flow of water out of the interstitial space into the capillaries, and then out of the cranium to the general circulation. Supporting this mechanism is evidence that osmotic diuretics are relatively ineffective when there is little brain parenchyma from which to extract water (39). Others claim that osmotic diuretics can actually decrease CSF production (23). Additionally, there may be an insignificant osmotically-driven flow of water back into the choroidal capillaries from the ventricles (21). Reduction in the total cerebral water can result in a decrease in ICP and an accompanying increase in cerebral perfusion pressure. Indeed, the purpose of osmotic therapy in most studies has been to decrease ICP, without necessarily achieving a reduction in ventricular size. A concern has been that prolonged use of osmotic diuretics may produce the so-called "rebound effect." This "effect" is an increase in interstitial brain water that can occur either when the osmotic diuretic enters the interstitial space or when other compensatory mechanisms shift water into the brain. Various osmotic diuretics have been used for the treatment of hydrocephalus, including isosorbide, mannitol, urea, and glycerol.

Isosorbide

Isosorbide is a derivative of sorbitol; it is an effective oral diuretic that has frequently been used to reduce ICP in patients with hydrocephalus. Its chief advantage over other osmotic diuretics (except glycerol) is its ability to be absorbed when given orally. Hayden et al treated 14 children with various types of obstructive hydrocephalus with isosorbide (1-3 gm/kg/dose) for up to 7 days (21). Continuous ventricular pressure monitoring was performed on all patients. Immediate decreases in ICP to pressures 19%-100% less than baseline were noted for up to 6 hours following a single dose and up to 18 hours following multiple doses of isosorbide. Rebound of ICP to 20%-40% of baseline ICP was noted in 6 of 14 patients; only 1 patient had rebound of ICP to levels greater than baseline. Significant dehydration and hypernatremia were noted in most patients treated for longer than 72 hours. Therefore, the authors only recommended isosorbide for short-term treatment of increased ICP due to hydrocephalus. They did *not* advocate indefinite use. Similar results were obtained in a follow-up study by the same authors involving 45 patients given 97 trials of isosorbide treatment (61). The mean duration of each trial was 4 days (1-54 days); the mean dose was 10 gm/kg/day (2-36 gm/kg/day). Treatment was effective in decreasing ICP in 54% of trials, ineffective in 40%, and intermediate in 6%. Significant toxicity was noted in 27% of trials and was most frequent in patients treated for 3-6 days. Treatment was more effective for communicating (66%), than for obstructive (33%) hydrocephalus. It was also most effective in patients with a cerebral mantle wider than 2 cm. The authors postulate that sufficient cerebral tissue is needed for isosorbide to be effective in decreasing ICP, since water is shifted from the parenchyma into the capillaries. They did not consider isosorbide's effect on reducing CSF production.

Lorber has advocated in a series of publications the use of isosorbide for *prolonged* periods to treat patients with various types of hydrocephalus (38, 39, 42). In his largest series, of 147 patients, 46 (31%) were treated with immediate shunt surgery (42). The remaining 101 (69%) infants were treated initially with isosorbide (mean dose 8 gm/kg/day). In 36% of these infants the rate of head growth fell and signs and symptoms of increased ICP improved, so that no shunt surgery was required. In 37% of patients isosorbide was effective for a period of time, but later shunt surgery was required. In 27% of patients there was not even transient benefit from isosorbide and all required shunt surgery.

Lorber followed his patients closely for many years, particularly regarding head size and cognitive function, and concluded that shunt surgery may control the rate of head growth in patients with hydrocephalus better than isosorbide treatment, but he found no correlation between eventual head size and intelligence. He did note that the worst intellectual outcomes were noted in patients who were immediately shunted, compared to those given isosorbide treatment initially. He attributes this poor outcome in the shunted group to the fact that patients in this group had more significant hydrocephalus than did those in the isosorbide group. Unfortunately, CT scanning was not performed routinely in this series of patients, so that no correlation of treatment to ventricular size could be made. Although many of the patients developed hypernatremia and dehydration during prolonged isosorbide treatment, no permanent sequelae could be attributed to these side effects.

Mannitol, Urea, and Glycerol

These osmotic diuretic agents have been used to treat only a few patients with hydrocephalus with the similar effect of either decreasing ICP or reducing ventriculomegaly. Hayden et al administered mannitol and urea to 2 patients with hydrocephalus while continuously monitoring their ICPs. With both drugs, ICP dropped rapidly from 50-100 mm H_2O to 0; this effect lasted only 3-4 hours, followed by a rebound of ICP above baseline (21). Taylor et al used glycerol (2 mg/kg every 6 hours) to treat infants with PHH (65). In 14 of 20 patients there was a halt in the progression of ventriculomegaly and in 5 patients ventriculomegaly totally resolved. Volpe notes that half of these infants may have had spontaneous resolution of transient hydrocephalus following IVH, so that the improvement in ventriculomegaly may not be entirely attributable to glycerol (69). Because of the small number of patients treated with these agents, little experience exists concerning their use in the treatment of hydrocephalus.

THERAPY TO INCREASE CSF ABSORPTION

Normally CSF is absorbed at the arachnoid villi at a rate of 0.02 ml/min in infants and 0.35 ml/min in adults. Hydrocephalus can develop when there is reduced CSF absorption at the villi. This is due to a decrease in absorptive surface area as a result of either *a*) blockage of the villi openings due to fibrin deposition along their passages, or *b*) compression of the villi due to increased hydrostatic pressure. The former can occur following subarachnoid hemorrhage (SAH) and bacterial meningitis. Experimental fibrinolytic therapies have been used in rare instances to treat hydrocephalus following these conditions. Compression of the villi due to hydrostatic pressure probably occurs in some degree in all forms of hydrocephalus. The theory is that increased ICP due to ventricular dilation leads to secondary collapse of a number of villi, resulting in decreased absorptive area and further ventricular dilation (56).

Thrombus-inhibiting and Fibrinolytic Therapy

Thrombus and fibrin deposition in the subarachnoid space over the cerebral convexity and in the cisterns following SAH and meningitis can lead to a significant decrease in CSF absorption resulting in hydrocephalus. Heparin inhibits thrombus formation, among other actions, but does not dissolve already-formed blood clots. Hyaluronidase, urokinase, and streptokinase act to lyse fibrin that has already formed. Steroids can slow the inflammatory response following SAH and meningitis, but do not inhibit fibroblast growth and collagen synthesis, both important steps in fibrin formation. Most therapeutic trials of thrombus inhibiting/fibrinolytic therapy have been conducted in experimental animals. There are only a few case reports of their use in humans with hydrocephalus.

Heparin

Heparin is composed of a group of heterogeneous mucopolysaccharides with a molecular weight of 12,000, which usually do not cross the blood-brain barrier into the CSF. Following SAH and meningitis there is a break in the barrier, thus potentially allowing the entry of heparin into the CSF. Blasberg et al injected heparinized and non-heparinized blood into the subarachoid cisterns of monkeys (8). They found that the non-heparinized animals had a marked reduction in CSF absorptive capacity that persisted for up to 3 months following the injections. The heparinized group had much greater, although not normal, CSF absorption, which normalized within 6 weeks. No mention is made regarding the prevention of hydrocephalus in these animals. There have been no studies regarding the systemic administration of heparin to achieve therapeutic levels in the

CSF. Further animal experiments are needed before heparin therapy to prevent hydrocephalus following SAH can be advocated in humans. Such testing should determine if systemically injected heparin can be given safely to animals following SAH to prevent hydrocephalus.

HYALURONIDASE, UROKINASE, AND STEROIDS

Hyaluronidase is an enzyme that hydrolyses hyaluronic acid, a component of fibrin. It has been used in animals to resolve peritoneal adhesions and in humans to treat hydrocephalus, mainly following tuberculous (Tb) meningitis. In one study, hyaluronidase was injected into the CSF of 15 patients with hydrocephalus following Tb-meningitis and their outcomes were compared to those of 15 patients with the same condition treated by shunt surgery (18). Hyaluronidase therapy was as good as shunt surgery in resolving or significantly improving the clinical condition of patients and no toxic side effects were noted. Unfortunately, no radiographic evidence of improvement in hydrocephalus is presented in this study. Julow treated 24 dogs with intrathecal urokinase after experimentally inducing SAH (33). He compared the degree of subarachnoid fibrosis in these animals as measured by electron microscopy to that found in a control group not given urokinase. Significantly less fibrosis was found in the urokinase-treated group of animals. No ventricular measurements were made during these experiments, so that it is not known whether urokinase therapy can prevent hydrocephalus following SAH. There have been individual case reports of the successful use of intrathecal steroids to prevent or alleviate arachnoiditis due to meningitis, SAH and subarachnoid Pantopaque (62). Yet after dexamethasone was injected intrathecally into 43 dogs with experimentally induced SAH, there was no prevention of subarachnoid fibrosis (34).

HEAD WRAPPING

It is known that a progressive increase in ICP from -100 to $+400$ mm H_2O results in increased CSF absorption at the arachnoid villi (7). At markedly increased ICP, the alternate pathway of transependymal flow is utilized for CSF absorption. Epstein et al applied these principles to the treatment of infants with hydrocephalus and normal or slightly increased ICP by compressive head wrapping (13). He later demonstrated that the ICP generated during such compression was 500-700 mm H_2O (12). One must assume that at these pressures transependymal CSF absorption occurred thereby decreasing ventricular volume. Routine CT was not available at the time of these studies to demonstrate transependymal flow radiographically. No short-term adverse side effects of this treatment were noted. Although several reports of compressive head wrapping for hydrocephalus have appeared since Epstein's original article (9, 54), improvement in neurosurgical and neuroradiologic-imaging techniques have relegated this treatment to the level of historical interest only (F. Epstein, personal communication).

SUMMARY

The medical treatment of hydrocephalus is not intended to replace shunt surgery. The latter still remains the initial treatment for rapidly progressive hydrocephalus, particularly when clinical signs of increased ICP are present. However, medical therapy can be useful for the temporary treatment of slowly progressive hydrocephalus. It is particularly useful in very young infants in whom shunt surgery may be risky; medical therapy can stablize hydrocephalus until shunt surgery can be performed more safely. In some cases of transient hydrocephalus, as can be seen following IVH in premature infants, medical therapy may be the sole treatment needed until hydrocephalus resolves spontaneously.

The type of medical therapy employed depends in part on the type of hydrocephalus, its etiology, and its rate of progression. Serial LPs are appropriate for treatment of communicating hydrocephalus following IVH, but have no effect in reducing obstructive hydrocephalus. Carbonic anhydrase inhibitors and osmotic diuretics are more useful as temporary treatments for hydrocephalus in certain situations. There are ongoing studies at Yale and Tufts Universities using carbonic anhydrase inhibitor therapy for neonatal PHH (C. Duncan and H. Gilmore, personal communication and unpublished data). Furosemide therapy may be too risky in very young infants due its potential to induce nephrocalcinosis. In older patients furosemide

may not have as great a risk for producing this side effect. Cardiac glycosides, heparin, and fibrinolytic therapy for hydrocephalus have rarely been used in humans; their routine use cannot be advocated at this time. Until a multicenter, controlled study is undertaken to compare the effects of medical therapies and shunt surgery, the choice of medical or surgical treatment for hydrocephalus will be dictated by the individual situation.

REFERENCES

1. Allan, W.C., Holt, P.J., Sawyer, L.R., et al. Ventricular dilation after neonatal periventricular-intraventricular hemorrhage: natural history and therapeutic implications. Am. J. Dis. Child, 136:589–593, 1982.
2. Allan, W.C., Dransfield, D.A., and Tito A.M. Ventricular dilation following periventricular-intraventricular hemorrhage: outcome at age 1 year. Pediatrics, 73:158–162, 1984.
3. Anwar, M., Kadam, S., Hiatt, I.M., et al. Serial lumbar punctures in prevention of post-hemorrhagic hydrocephalus in preterm infants. J. Pediatr., 107:446–450, 1985.
4. Amacher, A.L. and Wellington, J. Infantile hydrocephalus: long-term results of surgical therapy. Child's Brain, 11:217–229, 1984.
5. Bass, N.H., Fallstrom, Lundborg, P. Digoxin-induced arrest of the cerebrospinal fluid circulation in the infant rat: Implications for medical treatment of hydrocephalus during early postnatal life. Pediatr. Res., 13:26–30, 1979.
6. Bergman, I., Wald, E.R., Meyer, J.D., et al. Epidural abscess and vertebral osteomyelitis following serial lumbar punctures. Pediatrics, 72:476–480, 1983.
7. Bering, E.A., and Sato, O. Hydrocephalus: Changes in formation and absorption of cerebrospinal fluid within the cerebral ventricles. J. Neurosurg., 20:1050–1063, 1963.
8. Blasberg, R., Johnson, D., and Fenstermacher, J. Absorption resistance of cerebrospinal fluid after subarachnoid hemorrhage in the monkey: effects of heparin. Neurosurgery, 9:686–691, 1981.
9. Boltshauser, E. and Cavanagh, N. Hydrocephalus treated by compressive head wrapping. Arch. Dis. Child, 51:399, 1976.
10. Donat, J.F. Acetazolamide-induced improvement in hydrocephalus. Arch Neurol, 37:376, 1980.
11. Elvidge, A.R., Branch, C.L., and Thompson, G.B. Observations in a case of hydrocephalus treated with Diamox. J. Neurosurg., 14:628–633, 1957.
12. Epstein, F., Wald, A., and Hochwald, G.M. Intracranial pressure during compressive head wrapping in treatment of neonatal hydrocephalus. Pediatrics, 54:786–790, 1974.
13. Epstein, F., Hochwald, G.M., and Ransohoff, J. Neonatal hydrocephalus treated by compressive head wrapping. Lancet, 1:634–636, 1973.
14. Fishman, R.A. Cerebrospinal fluid in disease of the nervous system, ed. 1. pp. 23–28, 25, 37, 113–131, Philadelphia. W.B. Saunders, 1980.

15. Foltz, E.L. and Shurtleff, D.B. Five-year comparative study of hydrocephalus in children with and without operation in 113 cases. J. Neurosurg., *20*:1064–1068, 1963.

16. Goldstein, G.W., Chaplin, E.R., Maitland, J., *et al.* Transient hydrocephalus in premature infants: treatment by lumbar punctures. Lancet, *1*:512–514, 1976.

17. Gopinath, G., Bhatia, R., and Gopinath, P.G. Ultrastructural observations in experimental hydrocephalus in the rabbit. J. Neurol. Sci., *43*:333–334, 1979.

18. Gourie-Devi, M. and Satish, P. Hyaluronidase as an adjuvant in the treatment of cranial arachnoiditis (hydrocephalus and optochiasmatic arachnoiditis) complicating tuberculous meningitis. Acta Neurol. Scand., *62*:368–381, 1980.

19. Griebel, R., Khan, M., and Tan, L. CSF shunt complications: an analysis of contributory factors. Child's Nerv. Syst., *1*:77–80, 1985.

20. Hakim, S. and Adams, R.D. The special clinical problem of symptomatic hydrocephalus with normal cerebrospinal fluid pressure. Observations on cerebrospinal fluid hemodynamics. J. Neurol. Sci., *2*:307–327, 1965.

21. Hayden, P.W., Eldon, L.F., and Shurtleff, D.B. Effect of an oral osmotic agent on ventricular fluid pressure of hydrocephalic children. Pediatrics, *41*:955–967, 1968.

22. Hiratsuki, H., Tabata, H., Tsuruoka, S., *et al.* Evaluation of periventricular hypodensity in experimental hydrocephalus by metrizamide CT ventriculography. J. Neurosurg., *56*:235–240, 1982.

23. Hochwald, G.M., Wald, A., and Malhan, C. The sink action of cerebrospinal fluid volume flow. Arch. Neurol., *33*:339–342, 1976.

24. Huber, Z.A. Complications of shunt operations performed in 206 children because of communicating hydrocephalus. Zentralbl. Neurochir., *42*:165–168, 1981.

25. Hufnagle, K.G., Shadid, N.K., Penn, D., *et al.* Renal calcifications: a complication of long-term furosemide therapy in preterm infants. Pediatrics, *70*:360–363, 1982.

26. Huttenlocher, P.R. Treatment of hydrocephalus with acetazolamide. J. Pediatr., *66*:1023–1030, 1966.

27. Ivan, L.P., Choo, S.H., and Ventureyra, E.C. Complications of ventriculoatrical and ventriculoperitoneal shunts in a new children's hospital. Can. J. Surg., *23*:566–568, 1980.

28. James, A.E., Burns, B., Flor, W.F., *et al.* Pathophysiology of chronic communicating hydrocephalus in dogs (Canis familiaris). Experimental studies J. Neurol. Sci., *24*:151–178, 1975.

29. James, H.E. and Schut, L. Pitfalls in the diagnosis of arrested hydrocephalus. Acta Neurochir., *43*:13–17, 1978.

30. James, H.E., Walsh, J.W., Wilson, H.D., *et al.* Prospective randomized study of therapy in cerebrospinal fluid infection. Neurosurgery, *7*:459–463, 1980.

31. James, H.E., Bejar, R., Gluck, L., *et al.* Ventriculoperitoneal shunts in high risk newborns weighing under 2000 grams: a clinical report. Neurosurgery, *15*:198–202, 1984.

32. Jensen, F. Acquired hydrocephalus III. A pathophysiological study correlated with neuropathological findings and clinical manifestations. Acta Neurochirug., (WIEN) *47*:97–104, 1979.

33. Julow, J. Prevention of subarachnoid fibrosis after subarachnoid haemorrhage with urokinase: scanning electron microscopic study in the dog. Acta Neurochir., *51*:53–61, 1979.

34. Julow, J. The influence of dexamethasone on subarachnoid fibrosis after subarachnoid haemorrhage: scanning electron microscopic study in the dog. Acta Neurochir., *51*:53–51, 1979.

35. Kreusser, K.L., Tarby, T.J., Taylor D., *et al.* Rapidly progressive posthemorrhagic hydrocephalus. Am. J. Dis. Child, *138*:633–637, 1984.

36. Kreusser, K.L., Tarby, J.F., Kovnar, E., *et al.* Serial lumbar punctures for at least temporary amelioration of neonatal posthemorrhagic hydrocephalus. Pediatrics, *75*:719–723, 1985.

37. Laurence, K.M. The natural history of hydrocephalus. Lancet, *2*:1152–1160, 1958.

38. Lorber, J. The use of isosorbide in the treatment of hydrocephalus. Dev. Med. Child. Neurol., *14 (Supp 27)*:87–93, 1972.

39. Lorber, J. Isosorbide in the medical treatment of infantile hydrocephalus. J. Neurosurg., *39*:702–711, 1973.

40. Lorber, J. Isosorbide in the treatment of infantile hydrocephalus: observations with a new drug. Clin. Pediatr., *14*:916–919, 1975.

41. Lorber, J. Isosorbide in treatment of infantile hydrocephalus. Arch. Dis. Child, *50*:431–436, 1975.

42. Lorber, J., Salfield, S., and Lonton, T. Isosorbide in management of infantile hydrocephalus. Dev. Med. Child Neurol., *25*:502–511, 1983.

43. MacMahon, P. and Cooke, R.W. Hyponatremia caused by repeated cerebrospinal fluid drainage in posthemorrhagic hydrocephalus. Arch. Dis. Child, *58*:385–386, 1983.

44. McAllister, J.P., Maugans, T.A., Shah, V.M., *et al.* Neuronal effects of experimentally induced hydrocephalus in newborn rats. J. Neurosurg., *63*:776–783, 1985.

45. McCarthy, K.D., and Reed, D.J. The effect of acetazolamide and furosemide on cerebrospinal fluid production and choroid plexus carbonic anhydrase activity. J. Pharmacol. Exp. Ther., *189*:194–201, 1974.

46. Mantovani, J.F., Pasternak, J.F., Oommen, P.M., *et al.* Failure of daily lumbar punctures to prevent the development of hydrocephalus following intraventricular hemorrhage. J. Pediatr., *97*:278–281, 1980.

47. Maron, T.H. Carbonic anhydrase: chemistry, physiology, and inhibition. Physiol. Rev., *47*:595–781, 1967.

48. Mealey, J. and Barker, D.T. Failure of oral acetazolamide to avert hydrocephalus in infants with myelomeningocele. J. Pediatr., *72*:257–259, 1968.

49. Murata, T., Handa, H., Mori, K., *et al.* The significance of periventricular lucency on computed tomography: Experimental study with canine hydrocephalus. Neuroradiology, *20*:221–227, 1981.

50. Neblett, C.R., McNeel, D.P., Waltz, T.A., *et al.* Effect of cardiac glycosides on human cerebrospinal fluid production. Lancet, *2*:1008–1110, 1972.

51. Nyberg-Hansen, R., Torvik, A., and Bhatia, R. On the pathology of experimental hydrocephalus. Brain Res., *95*:343–350, 1975.

52. Page, R.B. Scanning electron microscopy of the ventricular system in normal and hydrocephalic rabbits. Preliminary report and atlas. J. Neurosurg., *42*:646–664, 1975.

53. Papile, L.A., Burstein, J., Burstein, R., *et al.* Post-hemorrhagic hydrocephalus in low-birth-weight infants: treatment by serial lumbar punctures. J. Pediatr., *97*:273–277, 1980.

54. Porter, F.N. Hydrocephalus treated by compressive head wrapping. Arch. Dis. Child, *50*:816–818, 1975.

55. Price, D.L., James, A.E., Sperber, E., *et al.* Communicating hydrocephalus. Cisternographic and neuropathologic studies. Arch. Neurol., *33*:15–20, 1976.

56. Raichle, M.E., Grubb, R.L., and Phelps, M.E. Cerebral hemodynamics and metabolism in pseudotumor cerebri. Ann. Neurol., *4*:104–111, 1987.

57. Reed, D.J. The effect of furosemide on cerebrospinal fluid flow in rabbits. Arch. Int. Pharmacodyn. Ther., *178*:324–330, 1969.

58. Rosenberg, G.A., Kyner, W.T., and Estrada, E. The effect of increased CSF pressure on interstitial fluid flow during ventriculo-cisternal perfusion in the cat. Brain Res., *232*:141–150, 1982.

59. Rubin, R.C., Hochwald, G.M., Tiell, M., *et al.* Hydrocephalus III. Reconstruction of the cerebral cortical mantle following ventricular shunting. Surg. Neurol., *5*:179–193, 1976.

60. Shinnar, S., Gammon, K., Bergman, E.W., *et al.* Management of hydrocephalus in infancy: use of acetazolamide and furosemide to avoid cerebrospinal fluid shunts. J. Pediatr., *107*:31–37, 1985.

61. Shurtleff, D.B. and Hayden, P.W. The treatment of hydrocephalus with isosorbide, an oral hyperosmotic agent. J. Clin. Pharmacol., *12*:108–114, 1972.

62. Smith, J.K. and Ross, L. Steroid suppression of meningeal inflammation caused by Pantopaque. Neurology, *9*:48–52, 1969.

63. Smith, K.M., Deddish, R.B., and Ogata, E.S. Meningitis associated with serial lumbar punctures and post-hemorrhagic hydrocephalus. J. Pediatr., *109*:1057–1060, 1986.

64. Sutton, L.N., Wood, J.H., Brooks, B.R., *et al.* Cerebrospinal fluid myelin basic protein in hydrocephalus. J. Neurosurg., *59*:467–470, 1983.

65. Taylor, D.A., Hill, A., Fishman, M.A., *et al.* Treatment of posthemorrhagic hydrocephalus with glycerol. Ann. Neurol., *10:297–300, 1981*.

66. Torvik, A. and Stenwig, A.E. The pathology of experimental obstructive hydrocephalus. Electron microscopic observations. Acta Neuropathol. (Berl), *29*:21–26, 1977.

67. Tschirgi, R.D., Frost, R.W., and Taylor, J.L. Inhibition of cerebrospinal fluid formation by a carbonic anhydrase inhibitor, 2-Acetylamino-1,3,4-thiazole-5-salonamide (Diamox). Proc. Soc. Exp. Biol. Med., *87*:373–376, 1954.

68. Vanucci, R.C., Hellmann, J., Dubynsky, O., *et al.* Cerebral oxidative metabolism in perinatal post-hemorrhagic hydrocephalus. Dev. Med. Child Neurol., *22*:308–316, 1980.

69. Volpe, J.J. Neurology of the newborn, p. 351, ed 2. Philadelphia, W.B. Saunders, 1987.

70. Weller, R.O. and Shulman, K. Infantile hydrocephalus: clinical, histological and ultrastructural study of brain damage. J. Neurosurg., *36*:255–265, 1972.

71. Weller, R.O. and Williams, B.N. Cerebral biopsy and assessment of brain damage in hydrocephalus. Arch. Dis. Child, *50*:763–768, 1975.

72. Weller, R.O. and Mitchell, J. Cerebrospinal fluid edema and its sequelae in hydrocephalus. Adv. Neurol., *28*:111–123, 1980.

73. Welch, K., Sadler, K., and Gold, G. Volume flow across choroidal ependyma of the rabbit. Am. J. Physiol., *210*:232–239, 1966.

74. Wikkelso, C., Andersson, H., Blomstrand, C., *et al.* The clinical effect of lumbar puncture in normal pressure hydrocephalus. J. Neurol. Neurosurg. Psychiatry, *45*:64–69, 1982.

75. Yashon, D. Prognosis in infantile hydrocephalus. Past and present. J. Neurosurg., *20*:105–111, 1963.

76. Young, H.F., Nulson, F.E., and Weiss, M.H. The relationship of intelligence and cerebral mantle in treated infantile hydrocephalus. Pediatrics, *52*:38–44, 1973.

CHAPTER 5

Techniques for CSF Diversion

J. GORDON McCOMB, M.D.

INTRODUCTION

To best manage hydrocephalus by cerebro-spinal fluid (CSF) diversion, the neurosurgeon should become familiar with a given shunting system and its peculiarities. However, the variety of shunting devices is so large and ever-changing that any discussion of such particulars in this chapter would rapidly become outdated (27). With some specific exceptions, most of the shunt hardware is roughly comparable, and it is discussed below in general terms.

The clinical experience from which the following comments are derived is overwhelmingly a pediatric one, but these techniques and equipment also apply, to a very large degree, to adults. Our series at the Childrens Hospital of Los Angeles is representative of most large pediatric neurosurgical services in that about half of its procedures are related to CSF diversion. Although operative shunt procedures may not seem as glamorous as other neurosurgical procedures, we can do great good by treating hydrocephalus correctly. To that end, shunt procedures should not be delegated to the most junior residents; they require the presence of an experienced neurosurgeon. Only with accumulated experience and meticulous attention to detail and technique can the complication rate associated with CSF diversion be kept low and further improved.

VENTRICULOSTOMY

General Considerations

Ventriculostomy is the placement of a drainage catheter via burr hole or similar technique into the ventricular system. It can be used to temporarily drain CSF in hopes that normal CSF absorption pathways will subsequently become reestablished, as in a patient with acute hydrocephalus secondary to intraventricular hemorrhage, or when a permanent shunting procedure would be inappropriate, as in a patient with infected CSF and hydrocephalus. Intraoperative ventriculostomy can improve exposure to lesions adjacent to the ventricular system, and intraoperative and postoperative intracranial pressure (ICP) can be monitored via the ventriculostomy, with CSF pressure reduced by drainage of CSF through the drainage catheter as needed.

The insertion site of the ventriculostomy is usually the frontal or posterior parietal region. The right side is usually chosen as it is rarely the dominant hemisphere. If one lateral ventricle is significantly more dilated than the other, ventriculostomy placement should be into the larger ventricle. Our preferred ventriculostomy insertion site is usually the frontal region, because the ventriculostomy can be placed with the patient fully supine so that the external landmarks are readily apparent, smaller ventricles may be cannulated more easily, the frontal region is easier to bandage, and there is little likelihood of the patient lying on the bandage or tubing. Also, if it is necessary to insert a permanent CSF diverting shunt, the frontal ventriculostomy is not in the operative field at the posterior parietal region, our preferred site for a permanent diverting system. The neurological risks are approximately the same for the frontal and parietal approaches, but a possible risk of frontal insertion is damaging the hypothalamic structures if the tubing is passed through the lateral ventricles and into the floor of the third ventricle. However, computerized tomography (CT) scans have shown on rare occasion that the catheter tip entered the hypothalamic region without clinical evidence of dysfunction.

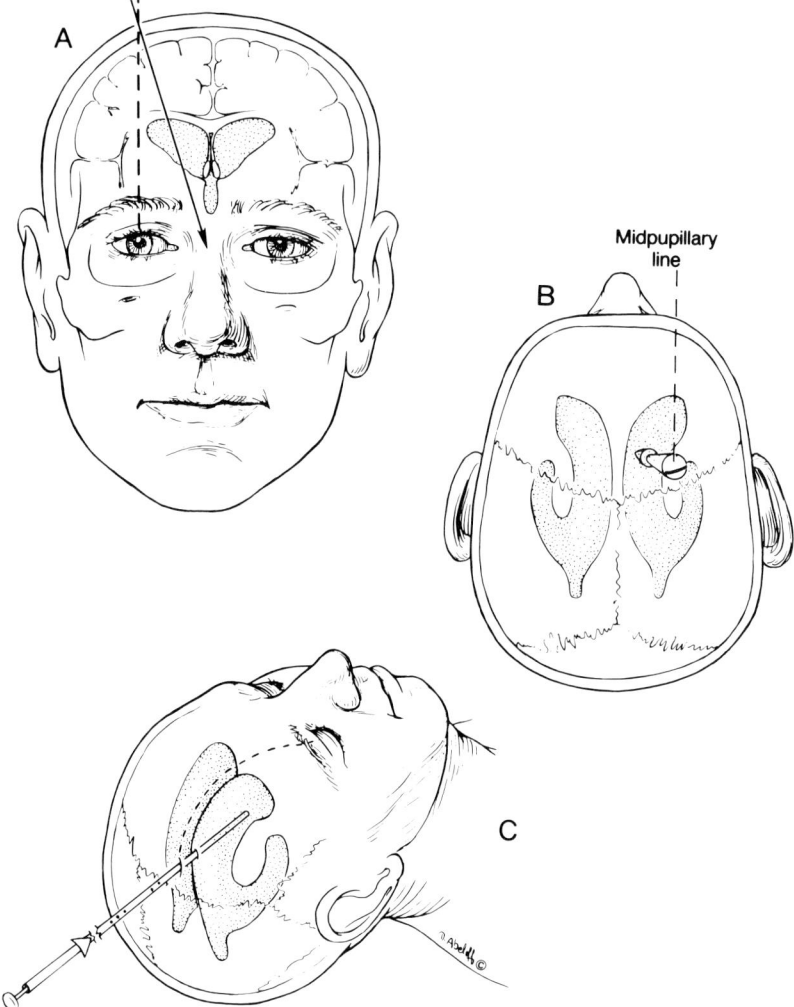

Figure 5.1.   Ventriculostomy placement. *A*) Frontal view, the catheter entry site is in the midpupillary line. Directing the tip of the catheter at the nasion ensures the greatest chance of the tubing entering the lateral ventricle. *B*) Catheter entry site in an older child or adult is approximately 1 cm anterior to the coronal suture. *C*) A 1 cm incision is made through the scalp. A hand or twist drill is used to make an opening in the skull.

Initial diagnostic studies are either CT scans or magnetic resonance imaging (MRI). If a question exists as to whether there is adequate communication between the two lateral ventricles, water-soluble contrast can be injected into the ventricular system once the ventriculostomy is in place. Small obstructing lesions in the region of the third ventricle, aqueduct of Sylvius, and fourth ventricle can be accurately outlined with a water-soluble contrast agent. Imaging modalities such as MRI have made this usually unnecessary.

Operative Technique

To minimize the possibility of infection, strict attention to aseptic technique is very important, whether the ventriculostomy is performed in the intensive care unit or in the operating room. Hair is removed for a considerable distance around the planned site. The skin is scrubbed with alcohol and a degreasing agent (such as Freon) and then well prepared with povidone-iodine (Betadine) solution.

At the site of planned incision, the skin is injected with lidocaine containing epinephrine.

In the child or adult, a linear incision 1 cm long is made 1 to 2 cm anterior to the coronal suture in the midpupillary line (Fig. 5.1*A* and 5.1*B*). The coronal suture itself is used as the entry site in the infant. A hand or twist drill may be used to make the opening through the skull. In the infant or young child in whom the skull is not thick, a smaller-diameter (5 mm) drill can be used. (In the older child or adult a larger hole is necessary, but it is easier to make the initial hole with a smaller bit followed by a larger one (7-8 mm) than by using the larger-diameter drill at the outset.) Keeping the head in the midline position with the face exposed will afford visibility of the external landmarks and thereby promote a more accurate placement of the ventriculostomy (Fig. 5.1*C*). A #11 blade is used to make certain that the inner table of bone has been adequately removed and to incise the dura mater, making it less likely that the dura mater will be stripped from the ventriculostomy entrance site, and decreasing the chance of an epidural hematoma.

For several years our unit has used a ventriculostomy tube modified by Holter-Hausner International Inc. (Bridgeport, PA) (Fig. 5.2) that has several advantages over others now available. The holes at the distal end of the catheter are covered with another layer of tubing containing longitudinal slits. The overlying slits make it less likely that the holes will be plugged with brain upon catheter entry. In addition, if the ventricles should collapse around the tubing, the holes are protected and have a greater chance of remaining patent. Markers on the tubing at 5 cm, 10 cm, and 15 cm intervals show the depth of penetration without the surgeon having to use a ruler. Tabs are bonded to the tubing and easily pass with it when making a subcutaneous tunnel. They are sewn to the scalp to prevent dislodgment.

The tubing is passed through the twist drill hole perpendicular to a tangent at the plane of the insertion site, with the tip directed toward the middle of the nose (Fig. 5.1*C*). Unless the ventricle is markedly dilated, it is usually entered 5 cm to 7 cm beneath the skin surface. The stylet is removed from the tubing and a curved, flanged trocar is attached to the end of the ventriculostomy tubing (after first checking to see that CSF will flow out the end), and secured with a suture (Fig. 5.3*A*). Using the catheter entry site, the trocar is pushed under the skin so it exits 6 cm or more from the point of insertion, thus creating a subcutaneous tunnel into which to tubing is pulled (Fig. 5.3*B*). Care is taken not to disturb the placement of the catheter tip within the ventricular system. The trocar is removed and patency is checked again to make certain that CSF is flowing freely from the tubing. A Luer-lok tip (Holter-Hausner International Inc., Bridgeport PA) is placed on the tubing along with a 1 ml tuberculin syringe to prevent any further loss of CSF (Fig. 5.3*C*). The Luer-lok tip is secured to the tubing with a suture. At the entry site the skin is closed with a single horizontal mattress suture. At the tube exit site, the tubing is secured to the skin by wrapping a suture affixed to the skin several times around the tubing and tying it securely, like a chest tube. The tubing is then brought anteriorly in a gentle loop and the two tabs are sutured to the skin to provide additional protection against dislodgment (Fig. 5.3*C*). The wounds are covered and taped. A tape mesentery is made for the tubing to firmly affix the catheter to the head (Figure 5.2*D*). Using a pressure (arterial type) tubing, the ventriculostomy catheter is connected to a transducer to monitor ICP and/or to drain CSF. With the ventriculostomy placed in such a location the patient has good head mobility and does not place any pressure on the tubing or dressing.

Complications

The most common complication of ventriculostomy is CSF infection. In a pediatric series of over 500 ventriculostomies, our CSF infection rate remains in the 2% to 3% range after an average monitoring of 7 days. This rate does not seem to be significantly related to the duration of placement, transient CSF leakage at the catheter site, or whether the ventriculosomy tubing was tunneled, but mainly to the patient's reduced resistance to infection. Tunneling has decreased the risk of CSF leakage, however. Our unit has had no wound infections. (Previously, approximately three quarters of our infections were from staphylococcal organisms; two thirds of these are *Staphylococcus epidermidis* and the other one-third from *S. aureus*. Prophylactic antibiotics have not been used routinely. Most infections are fairly easily cleared with the appropriate antibiotic therapy, especially if the ventriculostomy was removed.

A major complication would be a hematoma—epidural, subdural, or intraparenchy-

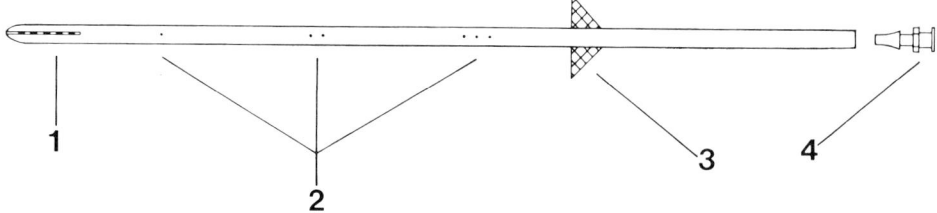

Figure 5.2. Ventriculostomy tubing has holes at the tip and is covered with slits (1) to protect the holes during placement and to diminish the chance that the brain could collapse around the holes and obstruct them. Marks on the tubing at 5, 10, and 15 cm (2) indicate depth of penetration. Tabs (3) to secure the tubing to the scalp are bonded to the catheter and easily pass with the tubing when making a subcutaneous tunnel. A Luer-lok (4) connector is attached.

mal—at the ventriculostomy site. This rare complication often has been associated with a known or unsuspected coagulation disorder. Our unit's rate of successful cannulation is 96%, and we have not encountered either a hemiparesis or hypothalamic dysfunction associated with ventriculostomy placement. When the ventricles are large they are easy to cannulate on the first attempt. If the ventricles are small the ventriculostomy is usually placed to monitor ICP, and only 2 passes are made at the ventricles. If the second attempt is not successful the tubing tip is left in the parenchyma. The wave form is dampened; however, it is still possible to accurately monitor ICP.

Seizures originating at the insertion site are another risk. As these patients often have one or more reasons to experience seizures it is usually not possible to ascribe seizures to ventriculostomy insertion unless electroencephalogram (EEG) tracings show epileptiform activity localized to the appropriate site.

EXTRACRANIAL CSF DIVERSION

General Considerations

Steady improvement in shunting hardware, associated with a progressive decline in shunt-related complication, have made extracranial shunting the procedure of choice when direct surgical removal of an obstruction is not feasible. The ideal shunt would be free of all complications and would drain the right amount of CSF continuously to maintain the appropriate normal physiological intraventricular pressure at all times. Such a goal is not obtainable with any currently available implanted mechanical device.

Extracranial CSF diverting shunts commonly used today include the ventriculo-peritoneal (VP), ventriculo-pleural (VPl), ventriculo-atrial

(VA), and lumbo-peritoneal (LP) varieties. Until the early 1970's the VA shunt was preferred for its high degree of success. VA shunts have been largely supplanted by VP shunts as the latter are technically easier to insert or distally revise and have fewer severe complications (18). Elective lengthening of the shunt can be avoided as enough tubing can be placed in the infant's abdominal cavity to allow for growth into adulthood, whereas VA shunts inserted in infants and children necessitate elective lengthening of the distal end at least once to maintain proper positioning of the tip in the atrium. The development of newer silicone elastomers and the insertion of enough tubing to allow the abdominal end to migrate freely about the peritoneal cavity have markedly diminished the problem of distal obstruction, the main factor which has allowed the VP shunt to supplant the VA variety; and on our service, less than a fraction of 1% of shunt insertions or revisions are of the VA type.

The other shunt that we now use for children over age 10 is the VPl type. It is almost as easy to insert the distal end of a VPl shunt into the pleural space is to insert tubing into the peritoneal cavity, and the prevalence and severity of complications are about the same. This shunt, however, cannot be used in infants and young children, whose pleural capacity frequently is inadequate and in whom hydrothorax would develop. Fortunately in the adolescent or adult patient this is rarely a problem.

Although this chapter will not discuss specific shunt hardware in detail, some general considerations should be kept in mind. All of the hardware should be seen easily in plain x-rays. Many of the earlier shunting devices were only visible at the very end of the ventricular and peritoneal/atrial catheters, and then often with some difficulty, making it impossible to

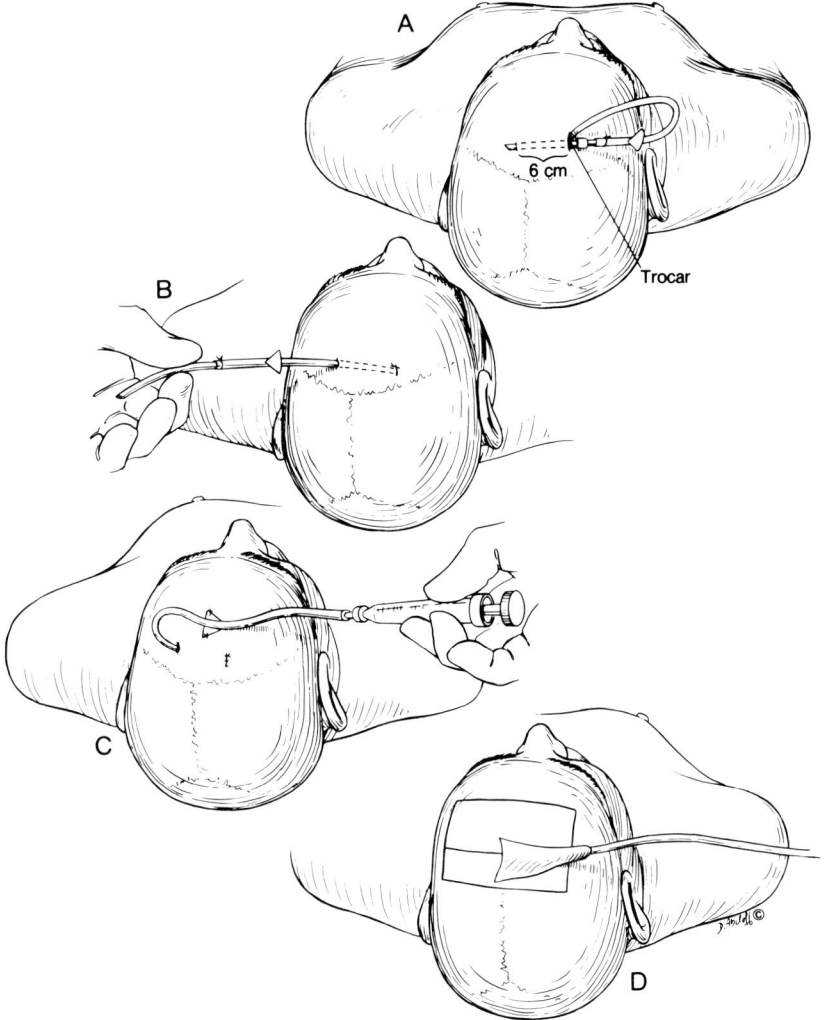

Figure 5.3. Ventriculostomy placement. *A*) Once the ventricle has been entered and CSF obtained, the stylette is removed and a trocar is attached to the end of the tubing and secured with a suture. The trocar is passed subcutaneously from the site of the initial incision and directed laterally to exit 6 cm or more distal to the entry site. *B*) The tubing is then pulled through the subcutaneous tunnel. The trocar is removed and the patency of the ventriculostomy tubing is confirmed. *C*) A Luer-lok connector is attached to the catheter and secured with a suture. A 1 cc tuberculin syringe is attached to prevent further loss of CSF. At the tubing exit site a suture is affixed to the skin, wrapped several times around the tubing, and tied. Tubing is gently curved anteriorly and tabs are sutured to the skin. Patency of the ventriculostomy is tested again. *D*) The area is taped.

see if the shunt was intact. This is becoming less of a problem as most manufacturers are producing radiopaque hardware so it is possible to see the shunt completely from one end to the other.

Although it is best to keep the shunt devices as simple as possible to minimize the chance of malfunction, our unit always places a reservoir in the system. We routinely tap the reservoir if there is any question as to function or infection of the shunt. The hair over the reservoir is shaved and prepped thoroughly with pre-packaged cotton-tipped applicators soaked with povidone-iodine (Betadine). The reservoir is tapped with a 25 gauge butterfly needle and the ventricular pressure is measured by holding up the tubing and noting the height to which the CSF rises. CSF can be aspirated and sent for analysis, or to relieve elevated ICP if indicated. Obstruction of the ventricular catheter, the most common source of shunt malfunction, is easily determined by tapping the reservoir as it will not be possible to aspirate CSF from the proximal end. The distal end of the shunt can also be tested for patency by injection of sterile saline. There are several different one-piece ventricular catheter reservoirs on the market that eliminate the need for a connector and markedly diminish the chance of separating the reservoir from the ventricular catheter, a problem with other systems—especially if the ventricular catheter is connected to the reservoir in the brain parenchyma well below the level of the calvarium.

Ventricular catheters have been made with various flanges at the tip in hope that the risk of proximal obstruction may be reduced; however, there is no good evidence that these are effective, and on the contrary, they can impede removal of the ventricular catheter if it needs to be replaced. A proximal valve with an open-end peritoneal tubing is preferred to shunts that have a slit valve at the peritoneal end, as this combination significantly reduces the frequency of distal obstruction. It is rare that we find it necessary to revise the open-ended peritoneal tubing because of occlusion.

Some evidence also suggests that a proximal valve may diminish the frequency of the slit-ventricle syndrome. We have not found it necessary to insert an 'anti-siphon' device with the use of a proximal valve (22). Using peritoneal tubing with a thick wall diminishes the chance that the tubing will kink, and once in place it facilitates shunt revision as the less-flexible tubing can be slid up and down the shunt tract to some degree. One manufacturer, using a thinner-walled tubing where kinking proved to be a problem, incorporated a wire coil within the tubing wall. This eliminated the kinking problem but has subsequently been associated with a higher frequency of viscus perforation because of catheter stiffness or exposure of wire if the catheter breaks. The steel used in the various valves and reservoirs is a non-magnetic stainless steel variety that does not preclude the use of MRI. The stainless steel does produce more of an artifact on both MRI and CT scans than those shunting devices using silicone elastomere only; however, it is rare that the artifact interferes with scan interpretation.

Skin incisions should be planned and outlined before draping. The superior sagittal sinus often is just to the right of midline in the posterior parietal region and may be a factor for the tendency to place the catheter entry site too far laterally. With growth of the skull in infants the shunt entry site will migrate laterally, resulting in a ventricular catheter with a definite curve. It is also important that the skin incisions be placed so that they are adjacent to, and not directly over, the shunt hardware, particularly in infants whose scalps are thin, to lessen the chance of wound breakdown and shunt infection. Also, thought must be given to possible future shunt revision when locating the incision and placement of various shunt components.

Permanent Shunt Placement

Whereas a frontal ventriculostomy insertion site is preferable, at this time our unit prefers the posterior parietal location for a permanent shunt. Disadvantages of the frontal approach include: a) more extensive hair shaving and scalp preparation, which can be of considerable concern to some patients and their families; b) tubing tunneled too closely to the ear makes it hard for the patient to wear glasses; c) an additional skin incision is needed in the posterior parietal region, as it is very difficult in infants and almost impossible in the adolescent or adult to tunnel the catheter from the frontal area to the distal entry site in one pass, and minimizing the number of skin incisions should lead to a lower shunt infection rate than is usual with a frontal approach.

The rationale for placing the tip of the ventricular catheter in the frontal horn, anterior to the foramen of Monro, is that the absence of choroid plexus tissue there reduces the chance that the ventricular catheter will be obstructed. However, a recent study reports that a frontally placed ventricular catheter has less chance of obstructing than a catheter placed properly in the frontal horn from a parietal entry site (1). More data are needed, and if substantiated our unit would switch to placing the shunts frontally in spite of the disadvantages noted above. An advantage to the frontal approach is the shorter distance and usually more easy access into the ventricle, a factor when the ventricles are not significantly enlarged. Our unit has not found access to be a particular problem with the posterior parietal approach if the projection of the frontal horn has been properly marked to provide good intraoperative orientation in directing the trajectory of the ventricular catheter toward the frontal horn. The posterior portion of the lateral ventricle usually dilates more readily than the frontal horn, making it easier to enter the lateral ventricular system there. Nonetheless, many published drawings show the ventricular catheter inserted well anterior to, and often inferior to, the desirable site of entry.

Operative Technique

Ventriculo-peritoneal Shunt

The patient is placed in the upper right corner of the table with the head turned to the left. This allows the anesthesiologist complete airway access (Fig. 5.4A). In infants, an esophageal stethoscope is used to avoid placing a stethoscope over the chest in the region of the operative field. A 'doughnut' made of any soft material is placed under the head. Padding is also inserted beneath the neck to make the angle between the head and chest as flat as possible, thereby making it easier to pass the tubing subcutaneously from the head to the abdomen. A rubber button stopper from a medicine bottle is placed on the patient's forehead in a position representing the anterior surface projection of the right frontal horn (Fig. 5.6B). The patient's skin is shaved and prepped with soap, alcohol, and a degreasing agent (such as Freon), and is well prepared with povidone-iodine (Betadine) solution. A thorough skin cleansing should reduce the skin bacterial count and presumably lower the risk of shunt infection. Excess povidone-iodine may be removed with more alcohol to ensure better adherence of a barrier drape to the skin, although this is not recommended by the manufacturer since it reduces the antiseptic iodophor residue on the skin. At this point the incisions are outlined with a skin marker to ensure proper orientation before draping. The skin may be sprayed with an antiseptic adhesive (such as Vidrape or Benzoin) to ensure better adherence of the barrier drape. Cloth towels are placed at some distance from the incision sites to prevent the barrier drape from sticking to the endotracheal tube, intravenous tube, etc. A barrier drape impregnated with povidone-iodine (Ioban) is placed over the exposed skin. Care is taken to ensure that the barrier drape adheres well to the skin, particularly at the incision sites. Paper drapes, impenetrable to liquid, are placed nearer to the proposed incision sites. A second layer of paper drapes is then placed around the patient and operating table. The skin is injected with a 0.25% lidocaine and 1:400,000 epinephrine solution to decrease bleeding.

A small curvilinear incision is made in the right posterior parietal area in the region of the projection of the occipital horn to the skin surface (Fig. 5.4). The scalp is reflected. A cruciate incision is made in the periosteum, which is elevated enough to allow a perforator to make a hole through the underlying bone (Fig. 5.5A). The hole is then enlarged using a small curette. The wound is next covered with a sponge moistened with either Ringer's lactate containing bacitracin or povidone-iodine and is covered with a towel to prevent contamination.

Attention is then directed to the abdomen, where a subxiphoid midline incision is made through the abdominal wall until the peritoneum is encountered and 2 4-0 absorbable sutures are placed into the peritoneum without opening this membrane. This eliminates hunting for the opening subsequently. (Although this author has no experience with the technique, some neurosurgeons place the peritoneal tubing percutaneously with a trocar, with only a slight increase in peritoneal complications and a slight reduction in operating time (25).)

A shunt tube passer is tunneled from the cephalic to the adominal incision without making any additional incisions along the pathway and the tubing implanted subcutaneously (Fig. 5.5B, 5.5C). The peritoneum is opened and the remainder of the tubing is placed into the abdominal cavity (Fig. 5.5D). For more than 10 years we have been using abdominal tubing 120 cm long, even in newborn infants, to eliminate the need to lengthen the shunt later. The tubing is flushed with Ringer's lactate containing bacitracin, thereby establishing that the distal end is patent with little resistance to flow. If a valve is to be used, it is inserted into the lumen of the proximal end of the tubing and affixed with non-absorbable 2-0 or 3-0 sutures (Fig. 5.5E).

Pinpoint cautery is used to make a hole through the exposed dura mater and underlying arachnoid and pia mater (Fig. 5.6A). If the cortex is thick the dural hole size is not critical; it should be big enough to allow the ventricular catheter to be introduced easily without resistance. If the cortex has been greatly thinned by the hydrocephalus, care is taken to ensure that the dural hole is slightly smaller than the diam-

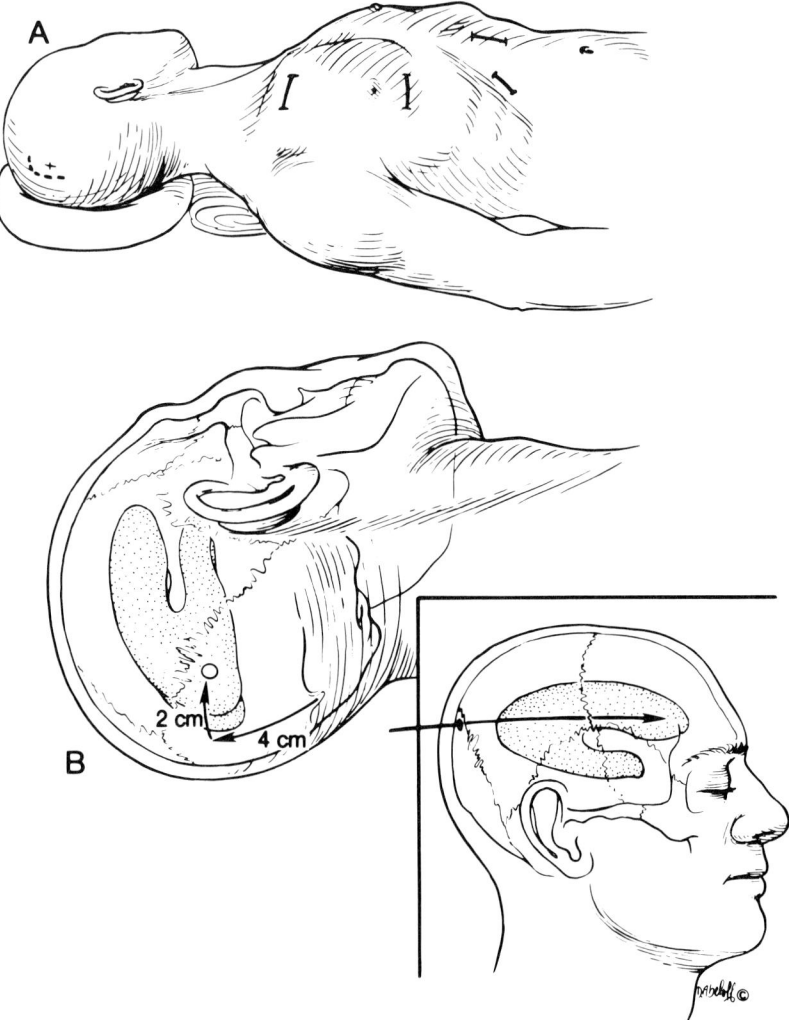

Figure 5.4.   Patient positioning and incision placement. *A)* Patient positioned for shunting procedure, head placed on a 'doughnut' to afford elevation and access to the posterior parietal region. Towels are under the neck. A curvilinear incision is made in the posterior parietal region midline to the site of catheter entry. The cephalic incision as outlined is adequate to revise the ventricular catheter or reservoir. For a ventriculo-peritoneal shunt a subxiphoid midline incision is preferred as it is not then necessary to cut through muscle. Otherwise use a right subcostal incision. For a ventriculo-pleural shunt make an incision at the 4th or 5th intercostal space in the midclavicular line just beneath the breast, or at the second or third intercostal space. For a ventriculo-atrial shunt a transverse incision is made midway between the mandible and clavicle extending anterior to the sternocleidomastoid muscle. *B)* Dilated ventricular system. In the average adult skull the projection of the occipital horn to the skin surface is about 4-6 cm above the inion and 2-3 cm lateral to the midline, the ideal site of catheter entry into the lateral ventricle.

eter of the ventricular catheter; this minimizes the possibility of CSF leakage around the entry site and a subcutaneous collection of fluid. Cortical bleeding is occasionally encountered, but it can be readily controlled with bipolar coagulation or direct pressure. From the CT or MRI scan and skull measurement the length of ventricular tubing needed to reach to the frontal

horn can be estimated accurately (Fig. 5.6*B*). In the older child and adult, a 12 cm ventricular catheter is usually adequate. After the ventricle is entered, CSF is obtained and sent for analysis of cells, sugar, and protein, and for culture (Fig. 5.6*C*). This is valuable for future reference. If indicated, CSF can also be obtained for cytology or biological marker examination.

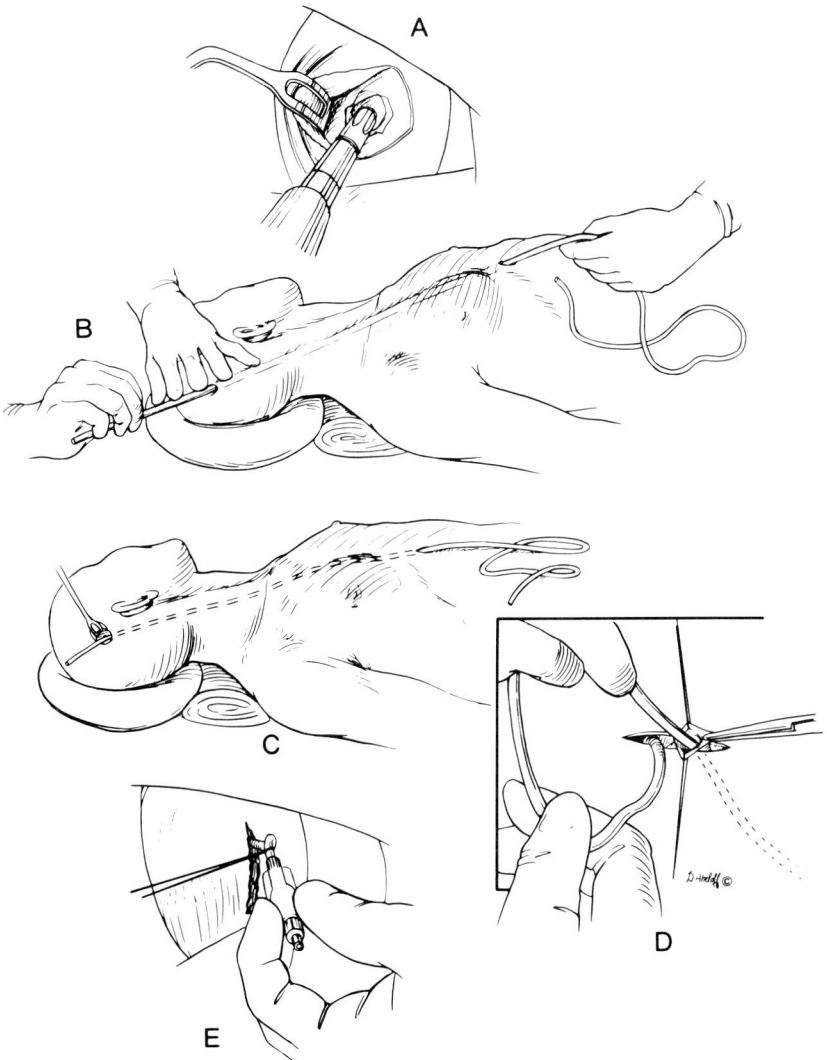

Figure 5.5. Ventriculo-peritoneal shunt. *A*) Scalp is reflected, periosteum elevated, and a burr hole placed. The dura mater is not yet opened. *B*) A subxiphoid incision is made in the abdomen. Abdominal wall layers are divided until the peritoneum is identified and tagged with 4-0 sutures but not opened. With trocar make a subcutaneous tunnel from the cephalic to the abdominal incision. *C*) Tubing is passed subcutaneously between the two incisions. *D*) Peritoneum is opened and the remainder of the peritoneal tubing is then placed into the abdominal cavity. The abdominal wound is covered. *E*) If valve is to be inserted, attach to the proximal end of the catheter and place under towels, minimizing exposure to the environment.

Care is taken not to drain an excessive amount of CSF, especially if the ventricles are large and the cortical mantle thin, as this increases the risk of subdural hematoma formation. If desired, an antibiotic may be injected into the ventricles. Our unit routinely injects 4 mg of gentamicin as a prepared 2 ml solution in a single disposable vial. The side arm of the ventricular catheter reservoir is then attached to the proximal end of the valve and secured with a 2-0 or 3-0 non-absorbable suture (Fig. 5.7). Attaching the side arm of the reservoir to the valve or peritoneal tubing immediately after placing the ventricular catheter diminishes CSF loss. If using separate reservoir rather than a one-piece ventricular catheter unit, it is better to attach the reservoir to the proximal end of the valve or peritoneal tubing before inserting the ventricular catheter. Once again, this minimizes CSF loss from the ventricles.

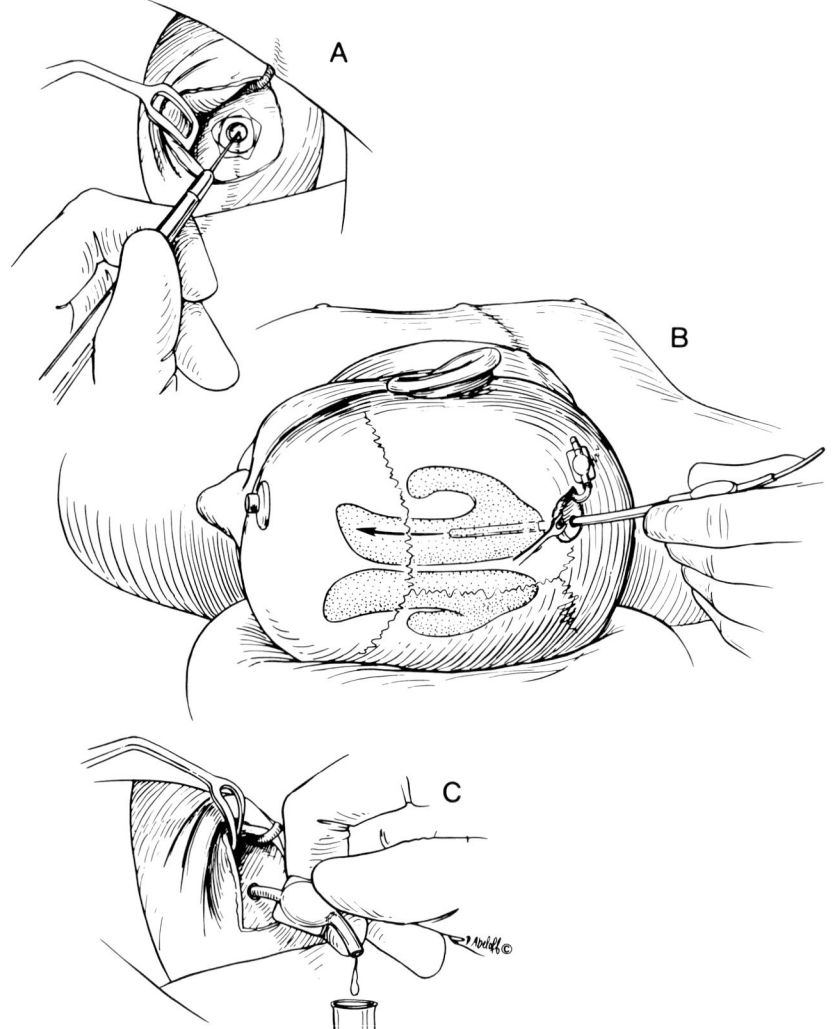

Figure 5.6. *A*) Pinpoint cautery is used to make a hole through the dura mater and the underlying pia-arachnoid. Control any cortical bleeding with bipolar coagulation. If the cortex is thick the dura opening should be made large enough to allow catheter entry without resistance. For markedly thin cortex make the dural opening slightly smaller than the diameter of the catheter to diminish the chance of leaking CSF. *B*) Placing the catheter tip in the frontal horn of a lateral ventricle should decrease the chance of obstruction by choroid plexus tissue. A button on the forehead to represent the projection of the frontal horn greatly aids in properly directing the catheter. *C*) With catheter in place CSF is obtained (for cell, sugar, and protein analysis, culture, and cytology or biogenic marker examination). A 1-piece ventricular catheter reservoir system is shown. If a separate reservoir is desired it should be attached to the proximal end of the valve before the ventricular catheter is placed.

The wounds are scrubbed with povidone-iodine solution followed by irrigation with Ringer's lactate containing bacitracin. The incisions are then closed using interrupted 3-0 or 4-0 absorbable sutures. The skin edges are approximated with tape such as Steri-strips.

The technique described can be used in the infant, child, or adult. Skin stitches are not used as the wounds heal better without them and there is no need to remove sutures; this is particularly a factor with an uncooperative patient. However, if there is any question about the integrity of the closure in regard to possible CSF leakage, a second layer of sutures placed in the skin is advisable. Sometimes this would also be done to control

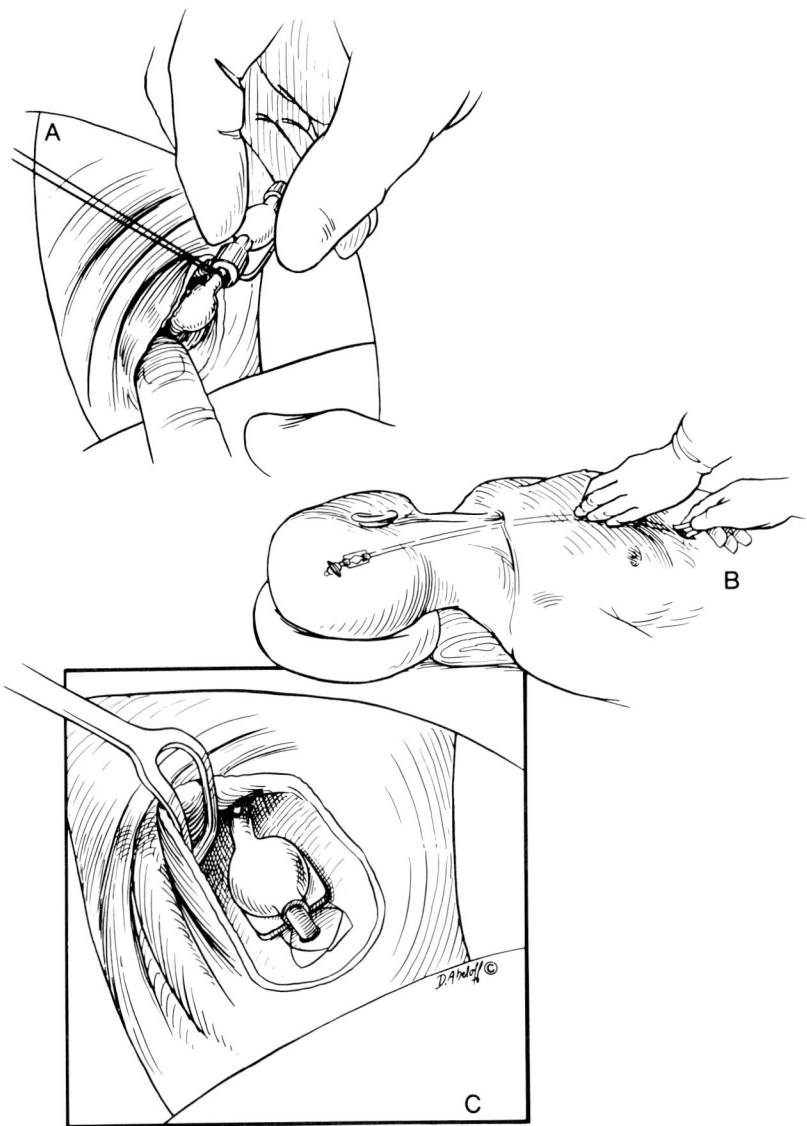

Figure 5.7. *A*) The side arm of the reservoir is attached to the proximal end of the valve with a nonabsorbable suture. *B*) From the abdominal incision pull the tubing (120 cm long) down to eliminate any possible kinks. Having no connectors in the peritoneal tubing eliminates a site for disconnection and in the child allows for tubing to migrate up the tract with little resistance. *C*) Reservoir and valve position at their final location. Hardware is directed away from the incision. Sutures are used to affix the reservoir to the pericranium to prevent dislodgement.

scalp bleeding at the termination of the procedure.

Ventriculo-pleural Shunt

As with a VP shunt, the cephalic incision is made first and the burr hole is placed. The wound is covered and attention is then directed to the chest wall.

For cosmesis, an incision approximately 3 cm long is made just below the breast in the midclavicular line (Fig. 5.4*A*). If the patient is obese or an incision higher on the chest wall is not objectionable, the site may be moved to the second or third intercostal space. The subcutaneous tissue, deep fascia, and pectoralis muscles are divided (Fig. 5.8*A*). It helps to wear a headlight to see more easily into the depths of the incision. The external and internal intercostal muscles are divided at the superior aspect of the lower of the 2 ribs of the intercostal space chosen. A self-retaining retractor placed between the 2 ribs opens the intercostal space even further (Fig. 5.6B). The parietal pleural is next seen with the lung beneath moving with respiration. The pleura is not opened at this point.

No additional incisions are necessary as the tubing is passed from the cephalic to the chest incision. Once the tubing is in its subcutaneous location the pleura is opened just enough to admit it (Fig. 5.8C). Twenty to 40 cm of tubing is inserted into the pleural cavity to provide redundancy and to ensure that the tubing will continually migrate in the pleural space. If the pleural opening is small it need not be sutured, but if larger it can be closed around the tubing with a 4-0 absorbable suture. Before the pleura is closed the anesthesiologist is asked to expand the lung to expel as much air as possible. This step can be repeated at closure of the first muscle layer. The remainder of this incision is closed as one closes the abdominal wall. A chest tube is unnecessary. A post-operative chest film is usually obtained.

Ventriculo-atrial Shunt

The cranial portion is handled in the same manner as a VP or VPl shunt.

An incision following a skin crease is made midway between the mandible and the clavicle (Fig. 5.9A). The platysma is divided and the anterior border of the sternocleidomastoid muscle is identified, dissected, and retracted posteriorly until the carotid sheath is located. The internal jugular vein is then separated from the common carotid artery and the vagus nerve. With further exposure the common facial vein is isolated for at least 1 cm before its entry into the internal jugular vein (Fig. 5.9B). If the common facial vein is not suitable as an entry site, the tubing can be placed directly into the internal jugular vein after placing a purse string suture in the vessel wall. The common facial vein is then ligated and tension applied to facilitate entry of the tubing. For control, temporary vascular clamps or loops are placed around the internal jugular vein proximal and distal to the entry site of the common facial vein (Figure 5.9C). A stick tie through the upper surface wall of the common facial vein is made proximal to the vein's entry into the internal jugular vein, and will be used subsequently to secure the atrial catheter. The length of atrial tubing needed to place the tip of the catheter to the appropriate position within the right atrium is estimated, and a reference suture or mark is placed on the tubing (Fig. 5.9B). The tubing tip is cut at a slight angle to facilitate its entry into the common facial vein. The tubing is filled with normal saline and clamped to prevent air from entering the atrium. The common facial vein is opened enough to admit the tubing and the catheter, which is advanced to the desired location.

As the length of tubing has only been estimated and it is also possible that the tubing could go into the wrong venous channels, it is necessary to confirm the catheter tip location. To do this a manometer is placed on the tubing and the pressure measured. If the pressure is low then the tip most likely is in the right atrium. If the pressure is over 10 cm of H_2O and pulsatile, the end is in the right ventricle, the tip having passed through the tricuspid valve. Pulling the tubing back should result in a pressure drop, indicating that the end now resides in the right atrium. In addition, there is usually a change in the P-wave of the electrocardiogram when the tubing tip is located in the right atrium. To be absolutely certain that the tip is in the position desired, the tubing should be injected with a contrast agent and visualized by intraoperative fluoroscopy. In the adult the midportion of the atrium is a satisfactory location for the catheter tip; in an infant or child it is best to position the end as low as possible within the atrium to allow for future growth.

The mark or suture on the tubing is noted in relation to its entry into the common facial vein so that final proper positioning is assured and to indicate that inadvertent movement of the tubing during subsequent steps in the operative procedure has not occurred (Figure 5.9E).

Whereas not placing a valve in a VP shunt is an option, it is imperative that a valve be placed in a VA shunt. The valve may be attached to the atrial catheter before or after the tubing is tunneled to the cephalic incision (Figure 5.9F). The stick tie through the wall of the common facial vein is now tied about the atrial catheter to secure its position. The remainder of the operative procedure is as described for a VP

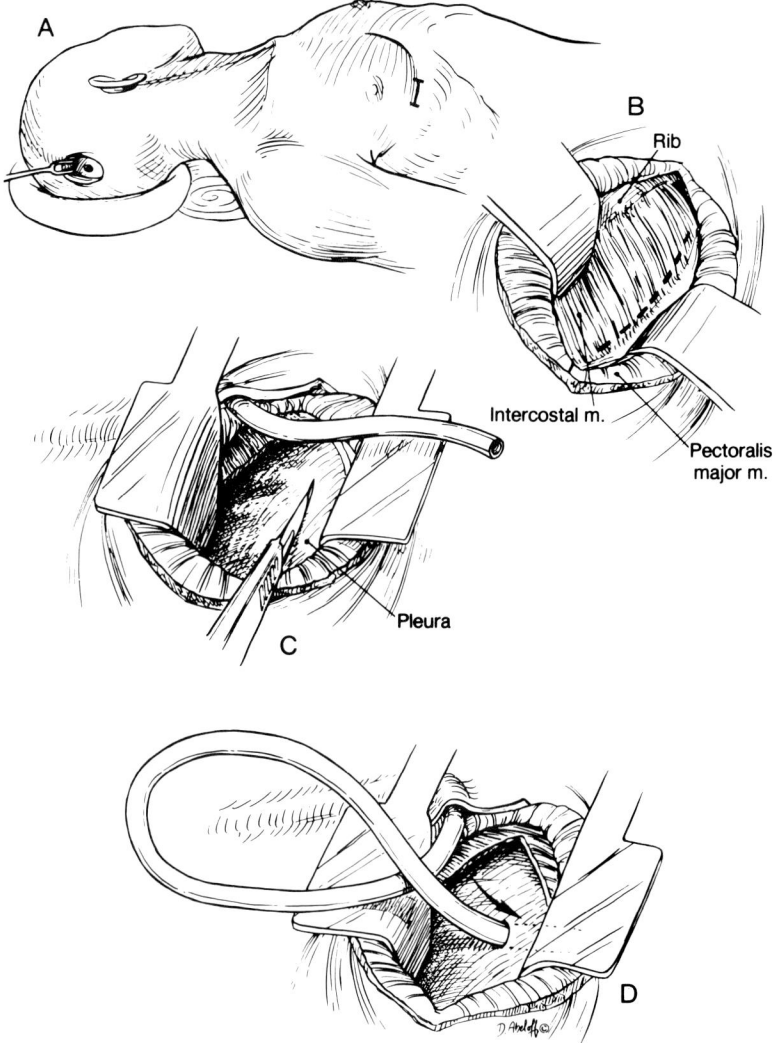

Figure 5.8. Ventriculo-pleural shunt. *A)* Incision is made just under the breast in the midclavicular line. Subcutaneous tissue and deep fascia are divided, followed by the pectoralis muscle. *B)* External and internal intercostal muscles are divided just above their attachment to the lowermost rib. A self-retaining retractor is used to spread the ribs. Tubing is passed subcutaneously as for a ventriculo-peritoneal shunt. *C), D)* A nick is made in the parietal pleura, and tubing 20 to 40 cm is placed in the pleural cavity. The wound is packed with moist gauze and covered with a towel. Other steps are as for a ventriculo-peritoneal shunt (Fig. 5.5.)

shunt. In contrast to a VP or VPl shunt, care must be taken to prevent more than a few cubic centimeters of air from entering the system lest air embolism result.

Biventricular Shunt

Biventricular shunts can be inserted in either the frontal or parietal locations (Fig. 5.10). If the frontal region is chosen the patient is positioned as described above. A 'doughnut' of increased thickness and of diameter less than the patient's head should be used to ensure adequate exposure to the down side-frontal region. With a parietal approach, the main potential problem is one of positioning. The patient is placed with the head face down to ensure good access to both posterior parietal regions. The torso is rotated to expose the right chest wall or right flank. In this position it is easy to make an incision in either the lateral chest wall for a VPl shunt or the right lower quadrant for a VP shunt. It is not possible to insert a VA shunt in this position.

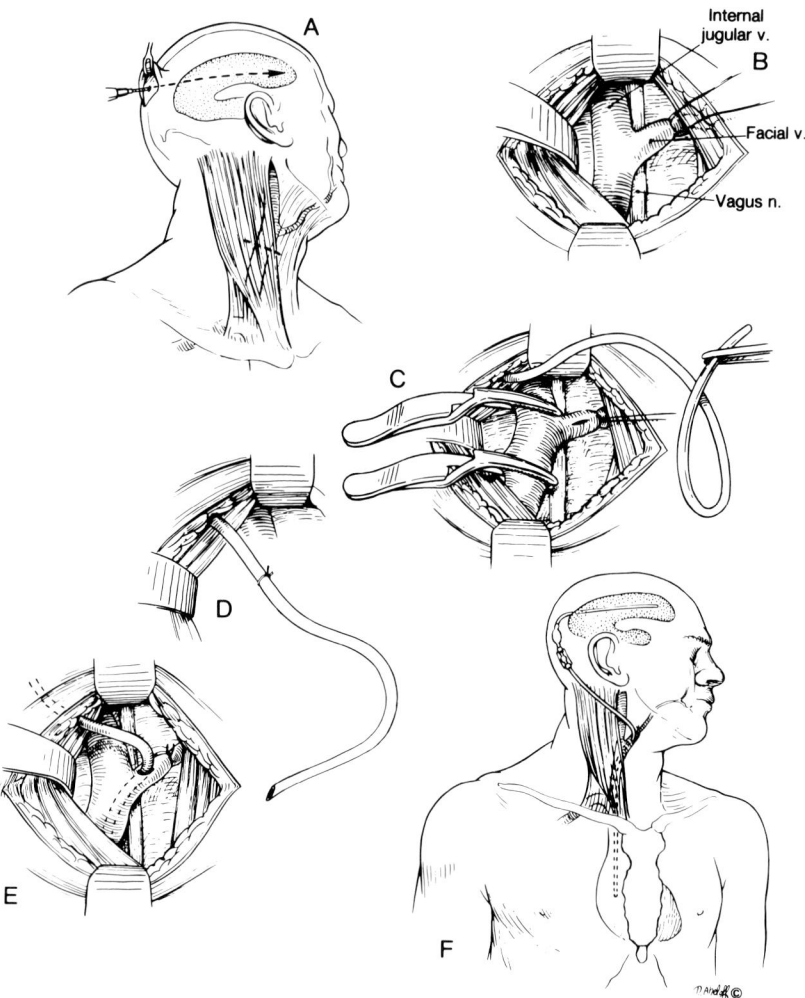

Figure 5.9. Ventriculo-atrial shunt. *A*) Head is placed as for a ventriculo-peritoneal shunt insertion. An incision is made midway between the mandible and the clavicle following a skin crease. The platysma is divided and the anterior border of the sternocleidomastoid muscle is identified, dissected, and retracted posteriorly until the carotid sheath is located. *B*) The internal jugular vein is separated from the common carotid artery and the vagus nerve. With additional dissection the common facial vein is isolated for at least 1 cm before its entry into the internal jugular vein. The common facial vein is ligated and put on tension. *C*) Temporary vascular clamps or vascular loops are placed about the internal jugular vein proximal and distal to the entry site of the common facial vein. A stick tie through the wall of the common facial vein is made proximal to its entry into the internal jugular vein. *D*) The length of tubing needed to place the tip of the catheter into the left atrium is estimated and a suture or mark is placed on the tubing for further reference. The tubing is cut at a slight angle to facilitate its entry into the common facial vein. The tubing is filled with normal saline and clamped to prevent air from entering the atrium. *E*) The common facial vein is opened and the tubing is advanced to the desired location. The catheter is checked for position manometrically and then with intraoperative fluoroscopy using injected contrast material. The mark or suture on the tubing is noted in relation to the catheter's entry into the common facial vein so that the correct final proper positioning is maintained and would indicate inadvertent movement of the tubing during subsequent steps in the operative procedure. *F*) The valve may be attached before or after the tubing is tunneled to the cephalic incision.

There are 3 options at this point. The 2 shunts can be treated independently, with 2 tubes tunneled to the pleural or abdominal cavity; the ventricular catheters can be connected by a Y or T connector proximal to the valve; or a valve can be placed just after the reservoir on each side and the 2 shunts be joined at a more distal location. What frequently happens, however, is that a catheter placed in one lateral ventricle initially drains both lateral ventricles sat-

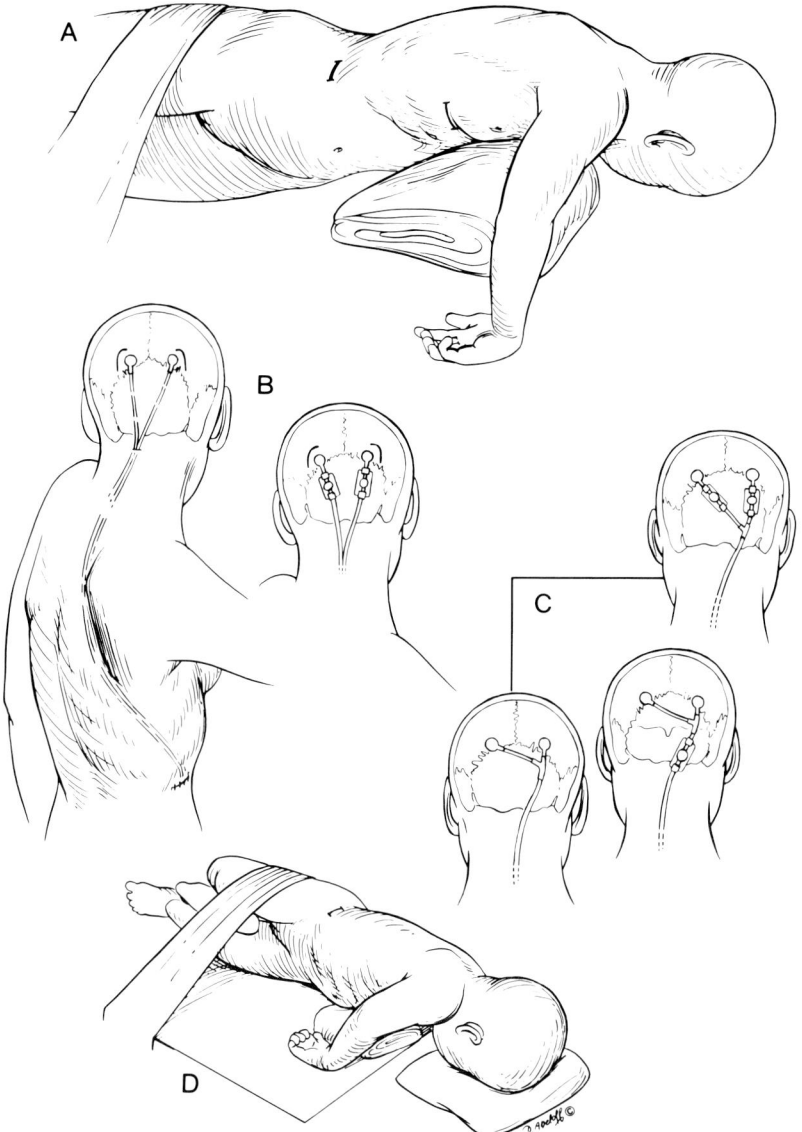

Figure 5.10. Biventricular shunt—parietal location. *A*) The patient is placed face down. The torso is rotated to expose the right chest wall or right flank for ready access to the right flank for a ventriculo-peritoneal shunt or the lateral chest wall for a ventriculo-pleural shunt. *B*) The 2 shunts can be treated independently with the 2 tubes tunneled to the abdominal or pleural cavity. The 2 independent systems can be used with or without valves. An incision in the neck is necessary, as it is not possible to tunnel the tubing from the posterior parietal region to the abdomen or chest in a single pass. *C*) If the 2 shunts are to be connected it can be done without a valve, or 1 valve, or with 2 valves. If no or 1 valve is to be used a T or Y connector can be placed in the sidearm of one of the reservoirs and the 2 shunts can be joined as diagramed. The other alternative is to place 2 valves in the system and join the system together with a Y connector at the neck incision. *D*) A child positioned for operation.

isfactorily. Then with subsequent tumor growth or scarring, the two lateral ventricles become isolated. The patient may become symptomatic with evidence of raised ICP or the problem may be detected by routine follow-up CT or MRI studies. At this point it becomes necessary to place a second ventricular catheter in the non-draining lateral ventricle. The choice in this situation is, as before, to connect the second ventricular catheter to the existing shunt or to insert an entirely separate new shunt. The technical ease of putting in a completely new second shunt is probably equivalent to connecting it into the existing shunt in the infant or child, but likely not in the adult. The advantage of 2 completely separate shunts is that they facilitate the diagnosis and treatment of a shunt malfunction and sometimes even infection. When designing the system and placing the incision, it is always best to consider that subsequent revision of the shunt might be necessary.

Lumbo-peritoneal Shunts

Both LP and VA shunts are very infrequently inserted on our service as the frequency of communicating hydrocephalus is much lower in the pediatric than in the adult population. A common indication for LP shunts in the adult is benign intracranial hypertension (pseudotumor cerebri), a condition rarely found in the pediatric age group. LP shunts require more operative manipulation for their insertion and revision, although newer percutaneous techniques appear to have solved this problem (16, 30). The complication rate for LP shunts appears similar to VP shunts, except that seizure activity secondary to catheter location is not a consideration for LP shunts. Previous reports of LP shunts in the pediatric age group have noted a high frequency of scoliosis, arachnoiditis, and radiculopathy, which may relate to hardware composition and sterilization and may be less applicable today (7, 19). Another complication of LP shunts in children is the development of the symptomatic "Chiari I" type of deformity, presumably due to the prolonged downward displacement of the inferior cerebellum into the foramen magnum following prolonged CSF drainage from the lumbar area.

The patient is positioned in the lateral decubitus position centrally on the table so that the surgeon and team have easy access to both abdomen and back. The back is moderately flexed to open the interlaminar spaces, and rolls are placed in the axilla and anterior to the abdomen to support the patient's position. A 'bean bag' positioning device, which can be formed to the patient and hardened by suction, is helpful (particularly in pediatric patients).

The lumbar catheter can be placed by percutaneous or open technique. The percutaneous technique employs a 14G Touhey needle through which the shunt tubing is passed. The ability of the tubing to pass through the needle

should be checked before shunt placement. A small incision is made in the low midline lumbar area through which the needle is advanced with its sharp tip parallel to the longitudinal fibers of the dura mater to allow more easy penetration. When CSF is encountered, the tip is advanced slightly, rotated 90° so that its opening is facing cephalad, and a predetermined length of tubing is threaded through the needle to place the catheter tip above the conus into the low thoracic region to avoid later traction on lumbar roots. If tubing will not pass easily, the needle tip is manipulated gently by angling the hub either in a cephalad or caudal direction and repeating the attempt. The needle is withdrawn over the tubing, with care taken not to pull back on the tubing until the needle is completely withdrawn to avoid inadvertently severing the catheter on the sharp needle tip. When CSF flow is observed from the catheter, it is tunneled around the flank to the peritoneum, and another opening is made to enter the peritoneal cavity. Occasionally, if the patient is obese or the subarachnoid space cannot be entered with certainty, a small partial laminotomy is necessary to open the dura under direct vision. Lateral approaches (such as rectus-splitting or McBurney-type incisions) to the peritoneal cavity are easier to carry out in this position than the strict midline approach advocated above. Available LP shunt systems have either distal slit valves or a variety of in-line systems, some of which require careful horizontal-vertical orientation where they are positioned. The systems can be tailored to a variety of valves using step-down connectors, which permit interchange of differing diameters of tubing and valve connectors. The shunt tubing should be anchored at the lumbar incision with a small silastic collar or other similar device to prevent its subsequent migration.

Complications

As the certain way to avoid shunt complications is not to insert one, it is first necessary to establish that the shunt is needed. Shunt complications can be divided into those that are common to all type of shunts and those that are unique to a particular type.

All shunts are subject to obstruction, disconnection, and infection. The frequency and location of obstruction and disconnection depend to a fair degree on the type of shunt hardware used. In general, the most frequent malfunction is occlusion somewhere within or around the ventricular catheter lumen. In the pediatric group, particularly those aged under 1 year, the most frequent cause of obstruction of the ventricular catheter is choroid plexus, ependymal, or glial tissue, which can grow into or surround the lumen. A distal slit-valve catheter is the next most frequent site of obstruction.

Another source of malfunction is disconnection, which can occur at any point in the system but is most often found where the various components are joined. Pressure-regulated valves can block, drain CSF at higher or lower than the intended pressure, or—rarely—allow retrograde flow, a concern in a VA shunt. Although it is possible that the higher the CSF protein, the more likely is valve obstruction, no definite relationship has been established. It is our unit's experience that, in the pediatric age group, the increased protein in CSF appears to be associated with more frequent ventricular catheter obstruction. As noted previously, the use of radiopaque materials for the entire length of the shunt is advocated, making it possible to determine the continuity of the shunting system on plain x-ray films. A reservoir in the system allowing access to the CSF is also helpful. By tapping the reservoir, pressure measurements can be made, the system's function can be ascertained, and CSF can be obtained for examination. If the adequacy of the shunt function is still in doubt after tapping the reservoir, imaging techniques that use contrast agents or radiopharmaceuticals can be used to determine patency.

Each type of shunting system has its own peculiarities that dictate how best to establish its functional adequacy. Most systems contain a pumping mechanism, either in the valve or the reservoir, which should test proper functioning. The response to pumping and proper functioning of the shunt may not correlate, with some shunts that do not pump normally functioning satisfactorily while others that pump normally are malfunctioning. If a shunt malfunction is suspected, our unit strongly advocates that response to pumping not be the sole criterion used to reach any definite conclusions.

The use of implanted materials always presents the risk of infection (9, 12). Prevention is preferable to treatment, and since most shunt infections probably occur at the time of insertion, revision, or (improper) tapping (28, 31), the use of meticulous aseptic surgical tech-

nique and possibly prophylactic antibiotics (14) are essential. They have reduced the risk of infection so that an operative infection rate of 5% or less should be the standard, with some centers reporting infection rates in the 1%-to-2% range (33, 36). A shunt infection may manifest itself with swelling and redness over a portion or all of the shunt tract as well as such generalized symptoms as peritonitis, with a VP shunt, or septicemia, with a VA shunt. Skin breakdown over the hardware and resultant shunt infection are seen more frequently in the infant. Proper incision and hardware placement and the use of low-profile and pliable materials should virtually eliminate this complication. Infection can be solely confined to the CSF in the ventricles and shunt, giving no external evidence other than a shunt malfunction. Initial infection rates for both VP and VA shunts are similar; however, the presence of a catheter within the atrium allows subsequent colonization during episodes of bacteremia (32). A VA shunt infection may lead to septicemia with subsequent systemic damage, whereas a VP shunt infection most commonly leads only to obstruction of the tubing's distal end. The most reliable way to confirm a shunt infection is to obtain several CSF samples from the shunt system (29). About half of the infecting organisms are *S. epidermidis*, a quarter are *S. aureus*, and the other quarter represents a wide variety of pathogens. The management of shunt infections still occasions considerable debate and is presented in Chapter 8 (17, 24, 35). Our unit's preference is usually for complete removal of the infected system with delayed replacement, as this has the best chance of success with the lowest morbidity and the shortest hospital stay. Delayed replacement usually necessitates CSF drainage intermittently via a reservoir or continuously by the establishment of an external ventricular drainage system.

Complications unique to VP shunts are ascites; pseudocyst formation; perforation of the viscus or abdominal wall; intestinal obstruction; spread of infection or neoplasm from the ventricles to the abdominal cavity; and a higher frequency of inguinal and umbilical hernias in infants (5). The use of a coiled spring inside the peritoneal catheter wall to prevent its kinking is responsible for most abdominal complications, as discussed above, and therefore its use is strongly discouraged. The length of tubing in the peritoneal cavity does not seem to be a factor in subsequent complications. Our unit has used a long length of peritoneal tubing for over 10 years even in the most premature neonates without any resultant complications. The complication that this author is aware of, but has never experienced, is that of producing a bowel obstruction in attempting to remove the peritoneal catheter from the cephalic incision. If the surgeon encountered increased resistance to removal of the tubing, and the tubing broke, it would be necessary to open the abdominal incision to remove the remaining tubing to ensure that the catheter has not encircled a segment of the intestine, constricting it and resulting in bowel obstruction and/or infarction. Use of longer tubing eliminates the need to lengthen the distal end of the shunt to accommodate growth. A problem noted recently is calcification and breakdown of the silastic elastomere in peritoneal catheters that have been in place for more than 10 years (6). The problem appears to be most noticeable in the neck region, and may be associated with repeated stress on the tubing by movement. With calcification the tubing becomes fixed to the surrounding fibrous tract and cannot migrate with growth. This has resulted in either disconnection of the shunt or fracture of the tubing. Interestingly, tubing within the peritoneal cavity does not show these changes. There have been occasional reports of malignant cells migrating to the peritoneal cavity via shunts for hydrocephalus, particularly of tumors associated with the primitive neuroectodural (PNET) variety. One preventive measure has been to insert a millipore filter in the shunt to block the tumor cells from advancing further (15), but unfortunately this filter rapidly develops increased resistance until the shunt malfunctions. Studies have shown that the frequency of tumor cells passed from the ventricular CSF to the abdominal cavity to produce viable tumor implants is small; the risk of extracranial CNS metastasis, particularly with PNET tumors, is no higher when CSF diverting shunts are present (23).

A complication of VPl shunts is fluid accumulation within the pleural cavity, particularly in the infant and child, but less so for the adolescent or adult. Hydrothorax is treated by moving the distal catheter to a site outside of the thoracic cavity. Once the source of incoming new fluid is eliminated, the fluid already in the pleural cavity is rapidly absorbed. Thoracentesis only need be done if the patient

is significantly symptomatic from respiratory distress.

Complications unique to vascular shunts involve the heart, lungs, and vasculature system, and include such major problems as subclavian and vena cava obstruction; mural thrombosis; bacterial endocarditis; cardiac arrhythmias; cardiac tamponade (secondary to perforation of the heart wall); embolization of the distal catheter into a pulmonary artery; and chronic pulmonary thromboembolization, which eventually produces pulmonary hypertension or cor pulmonale (8, 26). A complication of chronic low-grade shunt infection that is unique to VA shunts is nephritis, which develops from deposits of antibody-antigen and complement immune complexes in the glomeruli. The development of significant subdural fluid accumulations after ventricular shunting relates to the patient's age and the size of the ventricles, and the older the patient and bigger the ventricles the greater the risk for this complication, both during and after shunt insertion. Even a seemingly minor head injury may produce a significant subdural fluid accumulation if the shunted ventricles are large. The use of a higher pressure valve helps to reduce but does not eliminate this problem. If the subdural fluid collection is asymptomatic and relatively small, treatment is not necessarily indicated, but if a progressive increase in volume is documented and associated with clinical symptoms, it is necessary to drain the subdural fluid. This is best treated with a subdural peritoneal shunt without a valve to provide a pressure gradient across the cortical mantle between the two shunting systems.

The frequency of seizures in patients with shunted hydrocephalus is higher than can be attributed to hydrocephalus alone. This is substantiated by the finding of EEG abnormalities local to the site of shunt insertion. Previous reports have indicated that seizure frequency is much higher in shunts placed in the frontal location than in those in a parietal region, an observation that has come into recent question (3, 4, 13, 20, 21, 34). Whether prophylactic anticonvulsant treatment is needed and for how long is not clear, and is probably best decided on a case-by-case basis.

REFERENCES

1. Albright, A.L., Haines, S.J., and Taylor, F.H. Function of parietal and frontal shunts in childhood hydrocephalus. J. Neurosurg. 69:883–886, 1988.

2. Becker, D.P. and Nulsen, F.E. Control of hydrocephalus by valve-regulated venous shunt: avoidance of
complications in prolonged shunt maintenance. J.
Neurosurg. 28:215–226, 1968.

3. Copeland, G.P., Foy, P.M., and Shaw, M.D. The incidence of epilepsy after ventricular shunting operations. Surg. Neurol. 17:279–281, 1982.

4. Dan, N.G. and Wade, M.J. The incidence of epilepsy
after ventricular shunting procedures. J. Neurosurg.
65:19–21, 1986.

5. Davidson, R.I. Peritoneal bypass in the treatment of
hydrocephalus: Historical review of abdominal complications. J. Neurol. Neurosurg. Psychiatry
39:640–646, 1976.

6. Echizenya, K., Masaharu, S., Murai, H., et al. Miner-
alization and biodegradation of CSF shunting systems. J. Neurosurg. 67:584–591, 1987.

7. Eisenberg, H.M., Davidson, R.I., and Shillito, J. Jr.
Lumboperitoneal shunts. Review of 34 cases. J.
Neurosurg. 35:427–431, 1971.

8. Forrest, D.M. and Cooper, D.G.W. Complications of
ventriculo-atrial shunts: A review of 455 cases. J.
Neurosurg. 29:506–512, 1968.

9. Forward, K.R., Fewer, H.D., and Stiver, H.G. Cerebrospinal fluid shunt infections. A review of 35 infections in 32 patients. J. Neurosurg. 59:389–394,
1983.

10. Fox, J.L. and McCullough, D.C. The relative merits
of different shunting devices. In: Morley TP Current Controversies in Neurosurgery, edited by T.P.
Morley, pp. 671–685, Philadelphia, W.B. Saunders, 1976.

11. Fox, J.L., McCullough, D.C., and Green, R.C. Cerebrospinal fluid shunts: An experimental comparison
of flow rates and pressure valves in various com-
mercial systems. J. Neurosurg. 37:700–705, 1972.

12. George, R., Leibrock, L., and Epstein, M. Long-term
analysis of cerebrospinal fluid shunt infections. J.
Neurosurg. 51:804–811, 1979.

13. Graebner, R.W. and Celesia, G.G. EEG findings in
hydrocephalus and their relation to shunting procedures. Electroencephalogr. Clin. Neurophysiol.
35:517–521, 1973.

14. Haines, S.J. and Taylor, F. Prophylactic methicillin
for shunt operations: Effects on incidence of shunt
malfunction and infection. Child's Brain 9:10–22,
1982.

15. Hoffman, J.H., Hendrick, E.B., and Humphreys,
R.P. Metastasis via ventriculo-peritoneal shunt in
patients with medulloblastoma. J. Neurosurg.
44:562–566, 1976.

16. James, H.E. and Tibbs, P.A. Diverse clinical applications of percutaneous lumboperitoneal shunts. Neurosurgery 8:39–42, 1981.

17. James, H.E., Walsh, J.W., Wilson, H.D., et al. Prospective randomized study of therapy in cerebrospinal fluid shunt infection. Neurosurgery 7:459–463,
1980.

18. Keucher, T.R. and Mealey, J. Jr. Long-term results
after ventriculo-atrial and ventriculo-peritoneal

shunting for infantile hydrocephalus. J. Neurosurg.
50: 186–197, 1979.

19. Kusner, J., Alexander, E. Jr., Davis, C.H. Jr., et al.
Kyphoscoliosis following lumbar subarachnoid
shunts. J. Neurosurg. 34:783–791, 1971.

20. Laws, E.R. Jr. and Niedermeyer, E. EEG findings in
hydrocephalic patients with shunt procedures. Electroencephalogr. Clin. Neurophysiol. 29:325, 1970.

21. Leggate, J.L., Baxter, P., Minns, R.A., et al. Epilepsy following ventricular shunt placement (letter).
J. Neurosurg. 68:318–319, 1988.

22. McCullough, D.C. and Wells, M. Complications with
antisiphon devices in hydrocephalics with ventriculo-peritoneal shunts. Concepts Pediatr.
Neurosurg. 2:63–75, 1982.

23. McComb, J.G., David, R., Isaacs, and Hart, Jr. Ex-
traneural metastatic medulloblastoma during childhood. Neurosurgery 9:548–551, 1981.

24. McLaurin, R.L. Treatment of infected ventricular
shunts. Child's Brain 1:306–310, 1975.

25. Moss, S.D., Pattisapu, J.V., and Walker, M. Use of
the peritoneal trocar in pediatric shunt procedures.
Concepts Pediatr. Neurosurg. 8:23–28, 1988.

26. Nugent, G.R., Lucas, R., Judy, M., et al. Thrombo-
embolic complications of ventriculo-atrial shunts.
Angiocardiographic and pathologic correlations. J.
Neurosurg. 24:34–42, 1966.

27. Pudenz, R.H. The surgical treatment of hydrocepha-
lus-an historical review. Surg. Neurol. 15:15–26,
1981.

28. Renier, D., Lacombe, J., Pierre-Kahn, A., et al. Factors causing acute shunt infection: Computer analysis of 1174 operations. J. Neurosurg. 61:1072–
1078, 1984.

29. Schoenbaum, S.C., Gardner, P., and Shillito, J., Jr.
Infections of cerebrospinal fluid shunts: Epidemiol-
ogy, Clinical manifestations and therapy. J. Infect.
Dis. 131:543–552, 1975.

30. Selman, W.R., Spetzler, R.F., Wilson, C.B., et al.
Percutaneous lumboperitoneal shunt: Review of 130
cases. Neurosurgery 6:255–257, 1980.

31. Shapiro, S., Boaz, J., Kleiman, M., et al. Origin of
organisms infecting ventricular shunts. Neurosurgery 22:868–872, 1988.

32. Tabars, Z. and Forrest, D. Colonisation of CSF
shunts: Preventive measures. Kinderchir. 37:156–
157, 1982.

33. Venes, J.L. Control of shunt infection: Report of 150
consecutive cases. J. Neurosurg. 45:311–314,
1976.

34. Venes, J.L. and Dauser, R.C. Epilepsy following ventricular shunt placement (letter). J. Neurosurg.
66:154–155, 1987.

35. Walters, B.C., Hoffman, H.J., Hendrick, E.B., et al.
Cerebrospinal fluid shunt infection: Influences on
initial management and subsequent outcome. J.
Neurosurg. 60:1014–1021, 1984.

36. Welch, K. Residual shunt infection in a program
aimed at its prevention. Kinderchirurgie 28:374–
377, 1979.

CHAPTER 6

The Etiology and Management of Hydrocephalus in the Preterm Infant

ARTHUR E. MARLIN, M.D., and SARAH J. GASKILL, M.D.

INTRODUCTION

The treatment of posthemorrhagic hydrocephalus in the preterm infant has become a major problem in pediatric neurosurgery. Yearly, 35,000 infants weighing less then the 1 kg are born in the United States (32), and it is conceivable that with further progress in neonatology the number of viable preterm infants will increase. Among infants weighing less than 1500 g, 35% to 70% will sustain intraventricular hemorrhage (IVH) or germinal matrix hemorrhage, making this the most common serious neurological complication of the premature infant (33, 53). Of these children, 20% to 50% will go on to develop ventriculomegaly, either transient or progressive (16). This represents between 2,500 and 8,000 infants who will require treatment for posthemorrhagic hydrocephalus in the United States alone. These infants are frequently medically unstable; their treatment thus becomes a challenging problem. This chapter will discuss the management of hydrocephalus in the preterm infant and will review the predisposing factors and natural history of IVH.

ETIOLOGY AND PATHOPHYSIOLOGY

Several factors contribute to the premature patient's predisposition to IVH. The first is the basic anatomical structure of the germinal matrix. The hemorrhage arises from germinal matrix capillaries that have not yet fully developed and are readily susceptible to damage. Cells in this zone proliferate during the second to fourth months of gestation and then migrate to the cortex and deep nuclear structures. All neurons and glia are derived from the ventricular and subventricular zones of the germinal matrix.

The arterial blood supply to this region is from three main sources: *a*) the anterior cerebral artery through Huebner's artery; *b*) the middle cerebral artery through the deep lateral striates and penetrating branches; and *c*) the internal carotid artery through the anterior choroidal artery. The region drains via the internal cerebral vein. After this vein's formation from the terminal, choroidal, and thalamostriate veins, it makes a 180° turn at the caudate nucleus. It is possible that this anatomical arrangement predisposes to turbulence in blood flow and promotes platelet aggregation and vascular instability. The specific area of the hemorrhage will depend on the infant's gestational age and is based in part on the vasculature of the germinal matrix region and its developmental stage. The more premature the matrix, the more abundantly vascularized it tends to be. In infants of less than 28 weeks gestation the anterior choroidal and deep lateral striate artery territories are involved, and the hemorrhage tends to occur in the body of the caudate nucleus. In older infants, the head of the caudate is involved at the level of the foramen of Monro in the distribution of Huebner's artery. In mature or full-term infants, the choroid plexus is more likely to be the location of the hemorrhage (26).

Vascular factors crucial in the development of intraventricular hemorrhage also involve the nature of the periventricular capillaries. These vessels, which appear as a persisting immature vascular rete, cannot be distinguished as arterioles, capillaries, or venules; essentially they represent a layer of endothelium with little if any smooth muscle, no collagen, and no elastin (52). They are dependent upon oxidative metabolism and thus are readily injured by any hypoxic insult (50); they become more stable as the matrix is remodeled during maturation.

Another anatomical factor important in germinal matrix hemorrhage is the nature of the periventricular germinal matrix itself, which not only has a gelatinous consistency with poor support for blood vessels but also a high fibrinolytic activity, which may explain extension and dissection of the hemorrhage (18). Decreased tissue perfusion of this area occurs during the first few days after birth, coinciding with the peak frequency of hemorrhage. At this time the volume of the brain decreases, as does its turgor, and subatmospheric intracranial pressure (ICP) is common. This decrease in ICP parallels physiological dehydration and can be made worse by a hyperosmolar state or an anoxic insult.

Many changing factors in the premature newborn may predispose the patient to intraventricular hemorrhage. Cerebral blood flow, both its distribution and volume, seem to have great significance. There has been controversy, however, about whether the hemorrhage is related to high volume flow, a low volume flow, or a fluctuation in flow (23, 70).

The flow distribution to the germinal matrix from Huebner's artery, the anterior choroidal artery, and the lateral striates leads to a disproportionate amount of cerebral blood flow in the periventricular circulation during the period of greatest susceptibility. The caudate nucleus and cerebral cortex have a high flow; the subadjacent germinal matrix has a low flow. Changes in blood flow in these areas secondary to systemic change in blood pressure are well documented causes of IVH (19, 22, 26, 36, 69). Hypotension followed by rapid volume reexpansion is frequently the clinical context for hemorrhage (7, 8, 26, 57). Laboratory studies have investigated changes in cerebral blood flow in beagle puppies subjected to hypotension followed by rapid volume infusion (19, 20, 57). Following initial hypotension, increases in cerebral blood flow of up to 42% were documented. With reperfusion there were even further increases in cerebral blood flow, which could represent either a failure of the autoregulatory mechanism, or an early compensatory mechanism to provide adequate cerebral blood flow to meet oxygen requirements. The latter mechanism may simply represent the postischemic-hyperperfusion syndrome. Regardless of the mechanism, these increases in blood flow that occur with hypotension alone and then subsequently with reperfusion are potentially damaging to the unsupported, immature vasculature of the germinal matrix. It is reasonable to conclude that hypotension and rapid volume expansion each can precipitate an IVH.

The preterm infant is also susceptible to swings in systemic blood pressure. Increases in systemic blood pressure are then distributed to the cerebral vasculature. Moreover, obstruction of the venous sinuses will further exacerbate the increased pressure in the cerebral vasculature. For example, this can occur from deformation of the compliant skull during vaginal delivery. Any increase in blood pressure with a vasodilated microcirculation will increase or enhance the chances of germinal matrix hemorrhage (19, 22, 26, 36). These dramatic increases in blood pressure occur during apneic episodes, motor episodes, seizures, rapid eye movement sleep, exchange transfusions, rapid colloid infusions, and asphyxia. The preterm infant, while able to autoregulate cerebral blood flow, probably does so over an attenuated range (22), as normal systolic blood pressure is usually maintained below 60 mm Hg (29). In infants with a birth weight of 1500 g, the mean arterial pressure is only 40 mm Hg (47). This autoregulatory capacity is further impaired by asphyxia (35). Because asphyxia is so common in these infants, it seems reasonable to ignore autoregulation and consider cerebral blood flow as pressure-passive (9, 10, 35, 37). The most frequent series of events in the patient with IVH is asphyxia followed by hypoxia, hypercarbia, and acidosis, producing an increase in cerebral blood flow to an unstable vasculature.

A fluctuation in the flow pattern to the cerebral vasculature has also been implicated in IVH (70). Volpe believes that two basic cerebral blood flow patterns are demonstrable in these preterm infants—a stable pattern and a fluctuating pattern. The latter was correlated with the ensuing development of IVH. These fluctuations' etiology is respiratory in nature (55). This substantiates the role of both hypotension and hypertension in the development of IVH.

The hemorrhage itself can rupture into the ventricle or extend into the parenchyma. The mechanism for subsequent cerebrospinal fluid (CSF) obstruction may be a blood clot directly obstructing CSF flow. More commonly, an obliterating fibrosing arachnoiditis develops, resulting in a chronic and progressive hydrocephalus (27). The nature and mechanism of parenchymal extension of the hemorrhage are not yet clearly defined. A recent study of infants with germinal matrix hemorrhage or IVH found that a combination of three factors—hypothermia, low $PaO_2:FiO_2$ ratio, and severe bruising at birth—were predictive in 90% of infants who would subsequently develop intraparenchymal extension (64). There is debate whether the parenchymal extension of hemorrhage is true extension or concurrent hemorrhagic infarction (69). More recent evidence suggests that concurrent hemorrhagic infarction may indeed be the mechanism, or at least a separate, concurrently evolving lesion (52). This is likely to be associated with more serious tissue damage and subsequent morbidity. Intraparenchymal extension also correlates with an increased prevalence of porencephalic cysts.

BRAIN INJURY AND COMPLICATIONS OF IVH

Brain injury in intraventricular hemorrhage is caused by a myriad of factors: the hypoxic ischemic insult; increased ICP with decreased cerebral perfusion pressure; destruction of developing neural tissue; focal ischemia, and hydrocephalus. The hypoxic ischemic insult often precedes the bleed and may cause periventricular leucomalacia and selective neuronal injury (49, 66, 67). Increased ICP may be an important determinant of long-term brain injury as pressures in the range of 200-250mm/Hg may occur (70). Additionally, increases in CSF pressure have been shown to be associated with progressive ventricular dilatation and a much poorer neurodevelopmental outcome (1, 28, 51). This increase in CSF pressure, when associated with decreased blood pressure, causes a severe decrease in cerebral perfusion pressure and subsequent ischemia. Destruction of the developing neural elements from the bleed it-

self may cause focal motor lesions. Deficits in cerebral glia and myelinization are possible, as the germinal matrix cells are both glial and neuronal precursors. Extension or infarction may result in porencephalies or cystic lesions. Focal cerebral ischemia may be secondary to arterial vasospasm. While this is frequent in adults, it is not certain that it occurs in the preterm infant, but is suggested by doppler ultrasound studies of cerebral blood flow velocities in the anterior cerebral arteries (3).

Posthemorrhagic hydrocephalus will usually occur in the first to the third week after the hemorrhage. There is a good correlation between the severity of the hemorrhage and the possibility of developing hydrocephalus. The relation of the ventricular dilatation to the brain injury is difficult to evaluate. Whether the dilatation itself causes the damage or the dilatation is a response to earlier damage is uncertain. It is known that hydrocephalus as an isolated entity may be associated with a very good intellectual function, as, for example, in the hydrocephalus associated with myelomeningocele (42). The prognosis associated with intraventricular hemorrhage seems to be better correlated with the factors associated with the hemorrhage itself—for instance, hypoxia or acidosis—than with the hydrocephalus.

CLINICAL FEATURES

The hemorrhage itself can present as a catastrophic event or as a clinically silent phenomenon. It usually occurs within 48 hours of birth and will occur in the first 24 hours in 50% of the cases (51). Studies with chromium 50-labelled red blood cells show that the infant's median age at onset of hemorrhage is 38 hours (68); however, ultrasonography shows that 50% will occur in the first 24 hours (51). A later onset is not uncommon, especially following a secondary hypoxic insult such as pneumothorax.

The typical acute presentation is a catastrophic neurological deterioration that evolves in minutes to hours and consists of stupor, respiratory abnormalities, generalized tonic seizures, unreactive pupils, absence of extraocular movements, and flaccid paralysis, resulting ultimately in coma. The fontanelle will become full and the blood pressure and pulse will drop. Temperature instability is common, as are metabolic acidosis, a falling hematocrit, and abnormalities of glucose and fluid homeostasis. Acute hydrocephalus may occur. Many infants do not survive this event.

The subacute presentation is seen principally in an infant with a smaller hemorrhage that evolves over hours to days. There may be a subtle change in the state of consciousness, ranging from stupor to irritability. There is usually a decrease in tone and movements, both spontaneous and elicited. Abnormal eye movements, including skew deviation, downward drift, or loss of oculocephalic responses, have also been noted (70).

The silent hemorrhage is one diagnosed by ultrasonography. Retrospectively it may be associated with a decrease in hematocrit, decreased tone, poor activity, and impaired visual tracking, with development of roving eye movements.

DIAGNOSIS

The diagnosis of intraventricular hemorrhage and germinal matrix hemorrhage is primarily made by ultrasonography (6, 34). This technique has been most valuable in diagnosing and following the hemorrhage, the resulting ventriculomegaly, and cerebral damage. Because these children are very unstable, computed tomography (CT) has been less useful due to problems with transporting the infants.

Several investigational diagnostic modes have been used but do not have the reliability or the simplicity of ultrasonography. Transcephalic cerebral impedance, which is a measure of the resistance of the head and its contents to the flow of an alternating current, can help to diagnose the hemorrhage (61), depending upon gestational age. Alterations in intracranial fluid volume cause changes in the cerebral impedance, and a hemorrhage causes an increase in impedance. Unfortunately, this diagnostic technique is not readily available.

Evoked potentials may provide a functional measure of the integrity of the sensory pathways within the central nervous system and their disturbances by IVH, but their usefulness in this setting has not yet been defined.

Cerebral blood flow velocity as measured in the anterior cerebral arteries by a transcutaneous doppler technique has been shown to increase with pneumothorax, decrease with hydrocephalus, and then increase with the treatment of the hydrocephalus (3). Although this

technique may provide useful information, it remains investigational at present.

MANAGEMENT

When considering the management of any disease one must first consider the possibility of prevention. The prevention of a premature birth is not easily achieved, but it is possible to transfer mothers at risk to special birth centers. Transportation of the mother before delivery leads to a much lower prevalence of fetal IVH than transportation of the premature infant after delivery (70). Additional pre- and post-natal measures that have been attempted to decrease the risk of IVH include bethamethasone administration to the mother, which will decrease the severity of hyaline membrane disease and hence decreases the risk of IVH by improving the preterm infant's respiratory status (4). Other pharmacological means to prevent IVH have included the use of phenobarbital, ethamsylate, and indomethacin. In several institutions antenatal or postnatal phenobarbital protocols have produced marked decreases in IVH (11, 25, 59); however, this finding has not been supported by other similar studies (5, 71), and an adverse effect of phenobarbital on IVH has been documented by one investigator (56). The differences in results can be explained by variations in patient populations, time of initial dosing, administration route, and duration of therapy. Nevertheless, such wide variations in results make the decision to use phenobarbital or not a difficult one. A recent overview of the 9 previously published studies concluded that a risk-benefit ratio must be considered when using phenobarbital (11). They continue to support the use of phenobarbital for all infants weighing less than 1800 g when administered within 1 hour after birth. This is based on a reduction in the overall prevalence of IVH from 47% to 25% (the latter figure in infants less than 1500 g) in the 3-year period since the protocol was first instituted.

Ethamsylate is a capillary-stabilizing drug that is thought to reduce capillary bleeding by reinforcing the basement membrane through its action on the polymerization of hyaluronic acid and by increasing platelet adhesiveness. Its clinical usefulness is supported by a study that found a reduction in the frequency of germinal matrix hemorrhage in low birth weight infants (48). In this double-blind study of 70 infants, the use of 0.1 ml/kg of ethamsylate within 2 hours after birth and then Q6h for 4 days was found to decrease the risk of periventricular hemorrhage by 50% compared to the placebo group.

Indomethacin inhibits cyclo-oxygenase pathways of prostaglandin synthesis and prevents alterations (evoked by acute hypertension or asphyxia) in the cerebral microvascular permeability and morphology in experimental animals. It also lowers baseline cerebral blood flow and prevents rises in cerebral blood flow evoked by hypercarbia (45). In the beagle puppy model of IVH this has been proven effective in reducing hemorrhage (44, 46). The clinical studies to date, however, have not been as exciting as the experimental evidence (45).

Minimal stimulation protocols have been developed as a means of preventing sudden increases in blood pressure that might occur with patient handling as well as with the previously discussed rapid volume expansion, pneumothorax, seizures, and apnea. These protocols may aid in the prevention of IVH, but it is too early to evaluate their effectiveness.

MANAGEMENT OF HEMORRHAGE

When managing the IVH the first question to address is whether the child should be treated at all. The current debate over the decision to treat or not to treat is reminiscent of the debates about treatment of spina bifida 30 years ago. Since prognosis cannot be definitively determined and current studies (7, 15, 20), have conflicting reports, it seems reasonable to treat aggressively.

The 2 components of the issue are managing the acute IVH and managing the posthemorrhagic hydrocephalus. In the acute hemorrhage it is important to try to maintain cerebral perfusion pressure. Adequate systemic arterial pressure must be maintained because of the pressure-passive nature of cerebral blood flow, but too- aggressive therapy may change a small lesion to a large one. ICP should be lowered medically by decreasing the PCO_2, perhaps using furosemide, lumbar punctures, or ventricular taps (see below).

Evacuation of the hemorrhage is not feasible. Although early removal of the blood with ventricular catheters and subcutaneous ventricular reservoirs may prevent hydrocephalus, the catheter frequently clogs and only small amounts of blood can be removed. In a small number of patients in whom we have placed a subcutaneous ventricular reservoir early in the hemorrhage, it seems that fewer go on to develop progressive hydrocephalus, but we have not correlated our results with the size of the hemorrhage, and we do not believe that these attempts at early drainage of hematoma will make a significant difference (40).

MANAGEMENT OF POSTHEMORRHAGIC HYDROCEPHALUS

In the management of the posthemorrhagic ventriculomegaly or hydrocephalus, it is important to determine whether the ventriculomegaly is transient or progressive. Transient mild dilatation of the ventricular system in the neonate can occur without the clinical signs of increased ICP as cerebral volume and turgor diminish secondary to physiological dehydration. With the loss of weight and sodium, fluid redistributes in the body, so that more settles in the dependent parts. There is an increase in serum osmolality, with high urea levels after anoxia. In some preterm infants, up to 25% of total CSF volume may redistribute, and most excess fluid collects in the subarachnoid spaces over the convexities. Considerable ventriculomegaly can therefore occur before any increase in ICP or head circumference is noted. Transient ventricular dilatation is commonly seen with IVH. Because of its natural history of resolution, it is difficult to assess the results of early interventional treatments.

In 20% to 50% of patients with IVH, the ventriculomegaly will become progressive hydrocephalus with the clinical signs of increased ICP (16), and it is the management of this progressive hydrocephalus that has become a major problem in pediatric neurosurgery. Therapeutic options are pharmacological and surgical; the pharmacological options have usually been exhausted before the neurosurgeon is called.

Pharmacological Treatment

Pharmacological agents may include osmotic agents, loop diuretics, carbonic anhydrase inhibitors, and ATP-ase inhibitors.

Osmotic agents are used to increase serum osmolality and therefore decrease CSF production and brain water content. Isosorbide and glycerol and have been used. Both agents have produced moderate but transient benefits (62, 65), and the reduction in hydrocephalus has not lasted long enough to be significant. It must be remembered, however, that at times only short-term treatment is necessary. If the ventriculomegaly is transient, the agent's effect may be needed only until the ventricular dilatation has resolved.

The loop diuretics, such as furosemide, can be used for prolonged periods. They will decrease ICP, slightly decrease CSF formation, and promote CSF absorption (60). Once again, however, they do not provide a long-term solution to the problem.

Acetazolamide, a carbonic anhydrase inhibitor, has a transient effect in decreasing CSF formation. It can be used for days to weeks, but can cause significant electrolyte abnormalities, in particular a hyperchloremic metabolic acidosis. It is probably not as effective as furosemide. A theoretical objection to its use is that myelin contains carbonic anhydrase, and acetazolamide could therefore affect myelinization.

Acetazolamide and furosemide can be used in conjunction to provide an additive effect (60). One study showed that using this combined regimen in a selected population of patients with hydrocephalus of varied origin (including those with IVH), shunting was not necessary in more than 50% of cases (63).

Digoxin and other digitalis derivatives inhibit ATP-ase and will inhibit CSF formation; however, they will only do so for about 60 minutes and are not very effective long-term agents.

Treatment Procedures

Constrictive head wrapping has been proposed as a possible alternative to ventriculoperitoneal shunting (13). Its use in the neonate, however, has never been very effective because of the infant's delicate skin; the cranial distortion that it produces may be associated with hemodynamic changes and increases in ICP that may serve only to enhance the injury (14).

The most efficacious treatment modes of posthemorrhagic ventriculomegaly are CSF drainage procedures, the most common of which is serial lumbar punctures. For lumbar punctures to be effective the hydrocephalus must be communicating, and fortunately this is the most common type with IVH (58). In our practice the lumbar punctures are carried out by the neonatologists who frequently perform them for other reasons in these very small patients. The usual precautions should be taken—the 23 or 25 gauge spinal needle should have a stylet, and enough CSF—usually 3 ccs to 10 ccs—should be removed to control ICP. We have not measured pressures routinely, instead using fontanelle tension and degree of suture separation to determine amount of CSF removed and frequency of lumbar punctures. We have not used pre- and post-lumbar puncture ultrasound to determine whether the hydrocephalus is communicating and responding to this procedure because the vast majority of patients do have communicating hydrocephalus, but ultrasound can help in difficult cases. Many authors report the effectiveness of serial lumbar punctures (24, 54). They may promote CSF circulation both by removing blood products and highly proteinaceous fluid and by decreasing ICP. An unstable infant may be adversely affected by the positioning needed for lumbar puncture, and occasionally the lumbar theca cannot be entered successfully. There is also a body of literature that disputes the effectiveness of lumbar punctures (2, 38). In both these studies grade III and grade IV hemorrhages (53) were found to be especially resistant to preventing hydrocephalus through serial lumbar punctures.

If lumbar punctures and medical management fail, it seems reasonable to attempt to protect cortical mantle and normalize ICP by reducing ventricular CSF volume directly. While there are no definitive studies to indicate that this will produce a better outcome in the preterm infant, the study of Etches et al (15) suggests that this is the case. This goal can be achieved in several ways.

Serial ventricular punctures are a treatment alternative. The risks of cranial punctures include parenchymal, ventricular, or subdural hemorrhage. Multiple taps in the face of increased ICP may lead to the development of porencephalic areas. For this reason, serial ventricular punctures are not a satisfactory long-term option except in unusual circumstances.

External ventricular drainage (EVD) can be established with a single ventricular puncture to keep ICP consistently low. We have used any of the standard external ventricular drainage systems available on the market, making a small incision just anterior to the coronal suture, retracting the skin posteriorly, and entering the ventricle through the coronal suture. The drain is then tunnelled subcutaneously, either with the trocar supplied with the catheter or with a hemostat, to a site 3 cms to 5 cms distal to the incision. The drain valve is set 3 cm below the forehead level, since we believe that the normal intraventricular pressure in the premature infant is subatmospheric. We use prophylactic antibiotics just before placement of the drain and for the entire time the drain is in place. Rhodes reported a series of 38 patients in whom drainage was in place for an average of 21 days with an average of 1.8 drains required per patient (58). Ten patients died during this period, and of the total, the complications of placement were apnea (10%), hemorrhage (8%), and infection (6%). The drains were electively removed in 35% of the cases; however, 41% were removed or changed because of occlusion, and 13% became dislodged. Eleven percent were thought to be infected. EVD is a reasonable treatment option if the period before ventriculoperitoneal shunting is likely to be short, or if spontaneous resolution of the hydrocephalus might occur.

Early ventriculoperitoneal shunting in a series of patients has been reported by James et al. (31) and Boynton et al. (7). The surgery was carried out in a neonatal intensive care unit, however, and their infection rates were 26.9% if the patients were followed to discharge, 35.7% by 6 weeks following discharge, and 50% within 3 months of discharge. Of the group, 26.4% required revision during the nursery stay, and there were 142 revisions—1 to 11 per patient—in 34 patients within 3 months. We currently shunt these infants in the operating room, using a Leroy-type ventricular catheter and a distal open-ended catheter. Although we have not used a valve for the reasons cited above, a very small low pressure valve could be used in certain circumstances. We have had no complications putting the entire 90 cm catheter into the peritoneum, and have done so for many years. We are currently investigating the use of a portable disposable surgical isolation bubble in the intensive care unit in hopes of lowering the relatively high infection rates noted above while at the same time eliminating the need to transport these unstable infants to the operating room (Fig. 6.1).

Another drainage option is the use of a subcutaneous ventricular reservoir (Fig. 6.2A, B) (17, 39, 40, 41). Once again, the technique requires the performance of a single ventricular cannulation for catheter placement. The reservoir can then be aspirated percutaneously with a 27-gauge butterfly needle, daily or as frequently as necessary to control ICP and ventricular size. Placement of the reservoirs is performed in the neonatal intensive care unit with the infants on ventilators and in a warming unit (40). The right frontal and parietal regions are shaved and prepped. The skin just anterior to the coronal suture and over the parietal bone is infiltrated with normal saline. A semi-lunar incision is made anterior to the coronal suture, the skin is retracted to identify the suture, and the dura there is coagulated with a bipolar unit and incised. The reservoir is then placed into the right lateral ventricle, and the reservoir plug is secured with a 3-0 silk suture (certain catheter reservoirs come sealed or else have such tight-fitting plugs that this step may be omitted). The reservoir dome is placed underneath the skin over the parietal bone, and the incision is then irrigated with bacitracin solution and closed with 4-0 Prolene sutures that are left in place 2 weeks. It is very important the the incision be anterior to the catheter so that the catheter does not erode through the incision line. In a series of 38 patients reported by Gaskill et al. there were no infections in the reservoirs, no occlusions, dislodgements, or associated hemorrhages (17). Four patients eventually did not require a shunt and were weaned from their reservoir taps with mild to moderate ventricular dilatation. Initially 10 cc of CSF is removed with repeat sonography in 3 to 5 days to assess ventricular size. The amount and frequency of CSF aspiration is then changed empirically to keep the ventricular system, at most, mildly dilated. The frequency of sonograms varies with the patient's age and the length of time the reservoir is in place. It is more frequent initially if the ventriculomegaly does not respond readily. The amounts of CSF aspirated may vary between 5 cc and 10 cc every other day to up to 15 cc 3 times daily. If large amounts are being aspirated several times per day to control ICP, an early shunt should be considered. If the ventricular size and ICP are readily controlled, shunting is delayed until the patient is stable, gaining weight, and has resolved all the problems of its prematurity. The reservoir's major

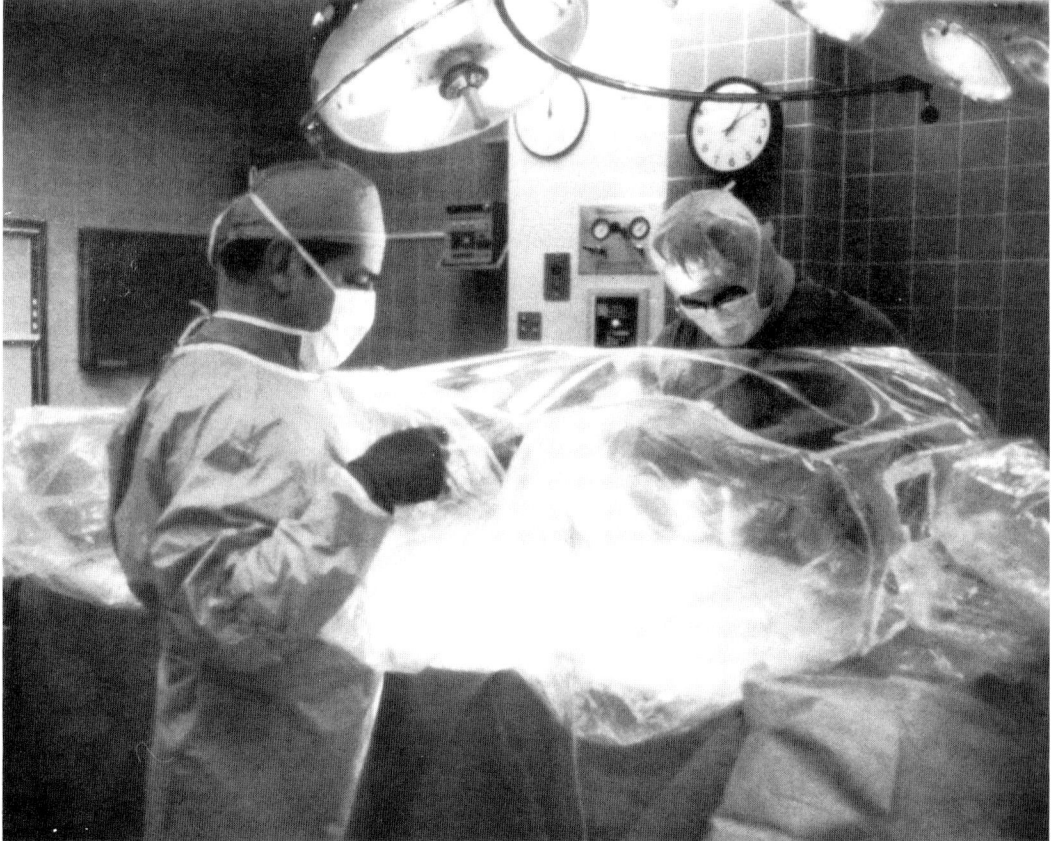

Figure 6.1. Portable disposable isolation bubble, which permits isolation of the infant from the ICU environment during placement of ventricular reservoir or shunt.

benefit is that it is simple, safe, and effective until the patient recovers from the problems of prematurity and is stable enough to go through a formal ventriculoperitoneal shunting procedure, if necessary. We have tended toward earlier reservoir placement and later shunting. The infection risk of subsequent shunting becomes quite acceptable, with a total shunt infection rate expressed per patient as 7% when followed to 6 months post-discharge (17).

Once the patient is ready for shunting and it has been determined that the ventriculomegaly or hydrocephalus is progressive, a ventriculoperitoneal shunt is the procedure of choice unless there have been significant abdominal complications, such as necrotizing enterocolitis, associated with the prematurity. In that case a ventriculoatrial shunt is used until the patient is larger. In general, low to very low pressure systems are recommended. It must be remembered that the CSF protein is typically high and that the normal

ICP in a premature child is atmospheric or subatmospheric. When the patient is on a respirator there is significant intraabdominal and intrathoracic pressure that may theoretically inhibit shunt function. A low pressure system that will handle the protein and elevation of the head of the bed to take advantage of the siphon effect may promote better shunt function.

PROGNOSIS

Despite many studies (7, 15, 70) it is difficult to make definitive statements about prognosis. Using the widely accepted hemorrhage classification of Papile (grade I hemorrhage is subependymal, grade II is intraventricular, grade III is intraventricular with ventricular dilatation, and grade IV is intraventricular with parenchymal extension [53]), a grade I hemorrhage generally has a good prognosis and a grade IV hemorrhage has a bad prognosis (Fig.

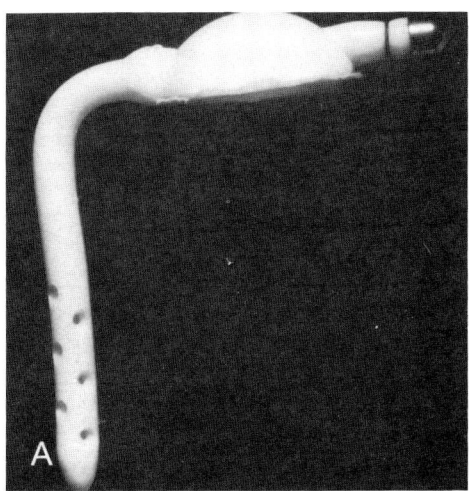
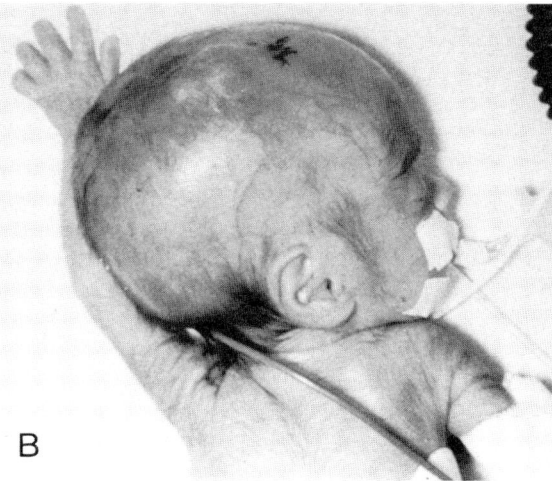

Figure 6.2. *A)* Right-angle ventricular catheter-reservoir used for intermittent ventricular aspiration. Recently-designed catheters have lower profiles and smaller bores. *B)* Infant in nursery with reservoir in place at coronal suture.

6.3). The prognosis for all bleeds will also depend upon the other factors of prematurity and the severity of the insults inflicted upon the developing brain. Volpe (70) correlated the short-term outcome of IVH in 800 cases as a function of the severity of hemorrhage. For mild hemorrhage he found a mortality rate of 15% and a progressive dilatation rate of 5%, for moderate 20% and 25%, for severe 40% and 55%, and for severe IVH associated with hemorrhagic intracerebral involvement 60% and 80% respectively. Regarding long-term outcome he reported on the prevalence of major neurological sequelae in 400 cases. For mild hemorrhage the risk was 15%, for moderate 30%, for severe 40%, and for severe hemorrhage with hemorrhagic intracerebral involvement 90%. Thus, the outlook for victims of significant IVH is not promising. Boynton et al. reported on 50 preterm infants requiring a ventriculoperitoneal shunt following IVH. The vast majority of their surviving patients had suffered grade III or IV hemorrhage; only 7 (18%) had normal developmental outcomes while 26 (60%) had multiple handicaps. In their series, grade IV hemorrhage or seizures was predictive of poor developmental outcome (7).

Etches et al. reported a study of 29 infants with birth weights of less than 2000 g who had been treated with ventricular shunts in the neonatal period for posthemorrhagic hydrocephalus. While the overall outcome was poor, they did find that neurodevelopmental outcome was improved when there were shorter intervals between diagnosis of hydrocephalus and definitive treatment (15). Their paper supports the notion that a definitive treatment regimen should be instituted promptly to achieve optimal neurodevelopmental outcome in these children.

Further studies are needed to provide more information about the etiology, natural history, prevention, and treatment of IVH.

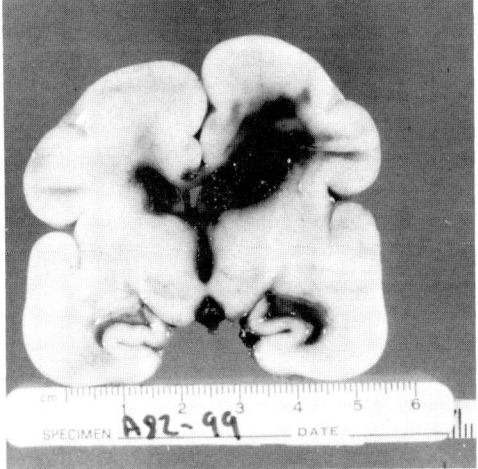

Figure 6.3. Post-mortem specimen from a premature infant with grade IV hemorrhage according to Papile's classification. Note extensive hemorrhage into brain parenchyma.

REFERENCES

1. Allan, W.C., Holt, P.S., Sawyer, L.R., *et al.* Ventricular dilatation after neonatal periventricular hemor-

rhage: natural history and therapeutic implications. Am. J. Dis. Child *136*:589–593, 1982.

2. Anwar, M., Kadan, S., Hiatt, I.M., *et al.* Serial lumbar punctures in prevention of post-hemorrhagic hydrocephalus in preterm infants. J. Pediatr. *107*:446–450, 1985.
3. Bada, H.S., Hajjar, W., Chua, C., *et al.* Noninvasive diagnosis of neonatal asphyxia and intraventricular hemorrhage by doppler ultrasound. J. Pediatr. *95*:775–779, 1979.
4. Ballard, P. and Ballard, R. Corticosteroids and respiratory distress syndrome: Status 1979. Pediatrics *63*:163–165, 1979.
5. Bedard, M.P., Shankaran, S., Slovis, T.L., *et al.* Effect of prophylactic phenobarbital on intraventricular hemorrhage in high-risk infants. Pediatrics *73*:435–439, 1984.
6. Bowerman, R.A., Donn, S.M., Silver, T.M. *et al.* Natural history of neonatal periventricular/intraventricular hemorrhage and its complications: sonographic observations. A.J.N.R. *5*:527–538, 1984.
7. Boynton, B.R., Boynton, C.A., Merritt, T.A., *et al.* Ventriculoperitoneal shunts in low birth weight infants with intracranial hemorrhage: neurodevelopmental outcome. Neurosurgery *18*:141–145, 1986.
8. Conner, E.S., Lorenzo, A.V., Welch, K., *et al.* The role of intracranial hypotension in neonatal intraventricular hemorrhage. J. Neurosurg. *58*:204–209, 1982.
9. Cooke, R.W.I., Rolfe, P., and Howat, P. Apparent cerebral blood flow in newborns with respiratory disease. Dev. Med. Child Neurol. *21*:154–160, 1979.
10. Daven, J.R., Milstein, J.M., and Guthrie, R.D. Cerebral vascular resistance in premature infants. Amer. J. Dis. Child *137*:328–331, 1983.
11. Donn, S.M., Roloff, D.W., and Goldstein, G.W. Prevention of intraventricular hemorrhage in preterm infants by phenobarbitone: a controlled trial. Lancet 2:215–217, 1981.
12. Donn, S.M., Goldstein, G.W., and Roloff, D.W. Prevention of intraventricular hemorrhage with phenobarbital therapy: now what? Pediatrics *77*:779–781, 1986.
13. Epstein, F.J., Hochwald, G.M., and Ransohoff, J. Neonatal hydrocephalus treated by compressive head wrapping. Lancet *1*:634–636, 1973.
14. Epstein, F.J., Wald, A., and Hochwald, G.M. Intracranial pressure during compressive head wrapping in treatment of neonatal hydrocephalus. Pediatrics *54*:786–790, 1974.
15. Etches, P.C., Chir, B., Ward, T.F., *et al.* Outcome of shunted posthemorrhagic hydrocephalus in premature infants. Pediatr. Neurol. *3*:136–140, 1987.
16. Fraser, R.A.R. and Patterson, R.H. Intracranial hemorrhage in unselected premature infants. Child's Brain *5*:574, 1979.
17. Gaskill, S.J., Marlin, A.E., and Rivera, S. The subcutaneous ventricular reservoir: an effective treatment for post-hemorrhagic hydrocephalus. Child's Nerv. Syst. *4*:291–295, 1988.
18. Gilles, F.H., Price, R.A., Kevy, S.V., *et al.* Fibrinolytic activity in the ganglionic eminence of the premature human brain. Biol. Neonate *18*:426–432, 1971.

19. Goddard, J., Lewis, R.M., Armstrong, D.L., *et al.* Moderate, rapidly induced hypertension as a cause of intraventricular hemorrhage in the newborn beagle model. J. Pediatr. *96*:1057–1060, 1980.
20. Goddard-Finegold, J., Armstrong, D., and Zeller, R.S. Brief clinical and laboratory observations: intraventricular hemorrhage following volume expansion after hypovolemic hypotension in the newborn beagle. J. Pediatr. *100*:796–799, 1982.
21. Deleted in proof.
22. Goddard-Finegold, J. Periventricular, intraventricular hemorrhages in the premature newborn: update on pathologic features, pathogenesis, and possible means of prevention. Arch. Neurol. *41*:766–771, 1984.
23. Goldberg, R.N., Chung, D., Goldman, S.L., *et al.* The association of rapid volume expansion and intraventricular hemorrhage in the preterm infants. J. Pediatr. *96*:1060–1063, 1980.
24. Goldstein, G.W., Chaplin, E.R., Maitland, J., *et al.* Transient hydrocephalus in premature infants: treatment by lumbar punctures. Lancet *1*:512–515, 1976.
25. Goldstein, G.W. and Donn, S.M. Periventricular and intraventricular hemorrhages. In: *Topics in Neonatal Neurology*, edited by H.B. Sarnat, pp. 83–108, New York, Grune and Stratton, 1984.
26. Hambleton, G. and Wigglesworth, J.S. Origin of intraventricular haemorrhage in the preterm infant. Arch. of Dis. in Child *51*:651–659, 1976.
27. Hill, A., Shackelford, G.D., and Volpe, J.J. A potential mechanism for early posthemorrhagic hydrocephalus in the premature newborn. Pediatrics *73*:19–21, 1984.
28. Kaiser, A.M. and Whitelaw, A.G. Cerebrospinal fluid pressure during post haemorrhagic ventricular dilatation in newborn infants. Arch. Dis. Child *60*:920–924, 1985.
29. Kitterman, J.A., Phibbs, R.H., and Tooley, W.H. Aortic Blood Pressure in normal newborn infants during the first 12 hours of life. Pediatrics *44*:959–968, 1969.
30. Kreusser, K.L., Tarby, T.J., Kovnar, E., *et al.* Serial lumbar punctures for at least temporary amelioration of neonatal posthemorrhagic hydrocephalus. Pediatrics *75*:719–724, 1985.
31. James, H.E., Bejar, R., Merritt, A., *et al.* Management of hydrocephalus secondary to intracranial hemorrhage in the high-risk newborn. Neurosurgery. *14*:612–617, 1984.
32. Larroche, J.C. Intraventricular hemorrhage in the premature neonate. Adv. Perinatol. Neurol. *1*:115–117, 1979.
33. Lee, B.C.P., Grassi, A.E., Schechner, S., *et al.* Neonatal intraventricular hemorrhage: a serial computed tomography study. J. Comput. Assist. Tomogr. *3*:483–490, 1979.
34. London, D.A., Carroll, B.A., and Enzmann, D.R. Sonography of ventricular size and germinal matrix hemorrhage in premature infants. A.J.N.R. *1*:295–300, 1980.
35. Lou, H.C., Lassen, N.A., Tweed, W.A., *et al.* Pressure passive cerebral blood flow and breakdown of the blood-brain barrier in experimental fetal asphyxia. Acta Paediatr. Scand. *68*:57–63, 1979.

36. Lou, H.C., Lassen, N.A., and Friis-Hansen, B. Is arterial hypertension crucial for the development of cerebral haemorrhage in premature infants? Lancet *1*(8128):1215–1217, 1979.

37. Lou, H.C., Lassen, N.A., and Friis-Hansen, B. Impaired autoregulation of cerebral blood flow in the distressed newborn infant. J. Pediatr. *94*:118–121, 1979.

38. Mantovani, J.F., Pasternak, J.F., Mathew, O.P., *et al.* Failure of daily lumbar punctures to prevent the development of hydrocephalus following intraventricular hemorrhage. J. Pediatr. *97*:278–281, 1980.

39. Marlin, A.E. Protection of the cortical mantle in premature infants with posthemorrhagic hydrocephalus. Neurosurgery *7*:464–468, 1980.

40. Marlin, A.E., Rivera, S., and Gaskill, S.J. The treatment of post-hemorrhagic hydrocephalus with the subcutaneous ventricular reservoir. In: Concepts in Pediatric Neurosurgery, Number 8, edited by A.E. Marlin, Basel, AG Karger, pp. 15–22, 1988.

41. McComb, J.G., Ramos, A.D., Platzker, A.C., *et al.* Management of hydrocephalus secondary to intraventricular hemorrhage in the preterm infant with a subcutaneous ventricular catheter reservoir. Neurosurgery. *13*:295–300, 1983.

42. McLone, D.G. Results of treatment of children born with a myelomeningocele. Clin. Neurosurg. *30*:407–412, 1983.

43. Ment, L.R., Stewart, W.B., Duncan, C.C., *et al.* Beagle puppy model of intraventricular hemorrhage. J. Neurosurg. *57*:219–222, 1982.

44. Ment, L.R., Stewart, W.B., Scott, D.T., *et al.* Beagle puppy model of intraventricular hemorrhage: randomized indomethacin prevention trial. Neurology *33*:179–184, 1983.

45. Ment, L.R., Duncan, C.C., Ehrenkranz, R.A., *et al.* Randomized indomethacin trial for the prevention of intraventricular hemorrhage in very low birth weight neonates. J. Pediatr. *107*:937–943, 1985.

46. Ment, L.R., Stewart, W.S., Duncan, C.C., *et al.* Beagle puppy model of perinatal cerebral infarction: regional cerebral prostaglandin changes during acute hypoxemia. J. Neurosurg. *65*:851–855, 1986.

47. Mondalou, H., Yeh, S.Y., Siassi, B., *et al.* Direct monitoring of arterial blood pressure in depressed and normal newborn infants during the first hour of life. J. Pediatr. *85*:553–559, 1974.

48. Morgan, M.E.I., Benson, J.W., and Cooke, R.W.I. Ethamsylate reduces the incidence of periventricular haemorrhage in very low birth weight babies. Lancet *2*:830–831, 1981.

49. Nwaesi, C.G., Pape, K.E., Martin, D.J., *et al.* Periventricular infarction diagnosed by ultrasound: a postmortem correlation. J. Pediatr. *105*:106–110, 1984.

50. Olendorf, W.H., Cornfor, M.E., and Braun, W.J. The apparent work capability of the blood-brain barrier: a study of the mitochondrial content of capillary endothelial cells in the brain and other tissues of the rat. Ann. Neurol. *1*:409–417, 1977.

51. Palmer, D., Dubowitz, L.M.S., Levene, M.I., Dubowitz, V. Developmental and neurological progress of preterm infants with intraventricular haemorrhage and ventricular dilatation. Arch. Dis. Child *57*:748–753, 1982.

52. Pape, K.E. and Wigglesworth, J.S. *Haemorrhage, Ischaemia, and the Perinatal Brain*. Philadelphia, J.B. Lippincott, 1979.

53. Papile, L., Burstein, J., Burstein, R., *et al.* Incidence and evolution of subependymal and intraventricular hemorrhage: a study of infants with birth weights less than 1500 grams. *J. Pediatr.* *92*:529–534, 1978.

54. Papile, L., Burstein, J., Burstein, R., *et al.* Posthemorrhagic hydrocephalus in premature infants: treatment by lumbar punctures. *J. Pediatr.* *97*:273–277, 1980.

55. Perlman, J. and Thach, B.T. Respiratory origin of the fluctuations in blood pressure associated with intraventricular hemorrhage in preterm infants. Pediatr. Res. *19*:357–361, 1985.

56. Porter, F.L., Marshall, R.E., Moore, J., *et al.* Effect of phenobarbital on motor activity and intraventricular hemorrhage in preterm infants with respiratory disease weighing less than 1500 grams. Am. J. Perinat. *2*:63–66, 1985.

57. Reynolds, M.L., Evans, C.A.N., Reynolds, E.O.R., *et al.* Intracranial haemorrhage in the preterm sheep fetus. Early Hum. Dev. *3*:163–186, 1979.

58. Rhodes, T., Edwards, W.H., Harbaugh, R.E., *et al.* External ventricular drainage for initial treatment of neonatal posthemorrhagic hydrocephalus. Presented at the Pediatric Section of American Association of Neurological Surgeons, Pittsburgh, 1986.

59. Ruth, V.L. Brain protection by phenobarbitone in very low birthweight prematures: a controlled trial. Klin. Paediatr. *197*:170–171, 1985.

60. Segae, M.B. and Pollay, M. The secretion of cerebrospinal fluid. Exp. Eye Res. [Supp.] *25*:127–148, 1977.

61. Siddiqi, S.F., Brown, D.Z., Dallman, D.E., *et al.* Detection of neonatal intraventricular hemorrhage using transcephalic impedance. Dev. Med. Child Neurol. *2*:440–447, 1980.

62. Salfield, A.W., Lorber, J., and Lonton, T. Isosorbide in the management of infantile hydrocephalus with glycerol. Arch. Dis. Child *56*:806–807, 1981.

63. Shinnar, S., Gammon, K., Bergman, E.W., *et al.* Management of hydrocephalus in infancy: use of acetazolamide and furosemide to avoid cerebrospinal fluid shunts. J. Pediatr. *107*:31–37, 1985.

64. Szymonowicz, W. and Wilson, F.E. Antecedents of periventricular haemorrhage in infants weighing 1250 g or less at birth. Arch. Dis. Child *59*:13–17, 1984.

65. Taylor, D.A., Hill, A., Fishman, M.A., *et al.* Treatment of posthemorrhagic hydrocephalus with glycerol. Ann. Neurol. *10*:297–301, 1981.

66. Trounce, J.Q., Fagan, D., and Levene, M.I. Intraventricular haemorrhage and periventricular leucomalacia: ultrasound and autopsy correlation. Arch. Dis. Child *61*:1203–1207, 1986.

67. Trounce, J.Q., Rutter, N., and Levene, M.I. Periventricular leucomalacia and intraventricular haemorrhage in the preterm neonate. Arch. Dis Child *61*:1196–1202, 1986.

68. Tsiantos, A., Victorin, L., Relier, J.P., *et al.* Intracranial hemorrhage in the prematurely born infant. J. Pediatr. *85*:854–859, 1974.

69. Volpe, J.J., Herscovitch, P., Perlman, J.M., *et al.* Positron emission tomography of the newborn: ex-

tensive impairment of regional cerebral blood flow with intraventricular hemorrhage and hemorrhagic intracerebral involvement. Pediatrics 72:589–601, 1983.

70. Volpe, J.J. Intracranial hemorrhage, periventricular-intraventricular hemorrhage of the premature infant. In: *Neurology of the Newborn*, Philadelphia, W.B. Saunders, pp. 311–361, 1987.

71. Whitelow, A., Placzek, M., Dubowitz, L., *et al.* Phenobarbitone for prevention of periventricular haemorrhage in very low birth-weight infants: a randomized double-blind trial. Lancet 2:1168–1170, 1983.

CHAPTER 7

Diagnosis and Treatment of the Slit Ventricle Syndrome

JEFFREY H. WISOFF, M.D., and FRED J. EPSTEIN, M.D.

INTRODUCTION

Since the introduction of the Spitz-Holter valve in 1952 (23) hydrocephalic children have been treated with a variety of shunting procedures. Routine postoperative computerized tomography (CT) demonstrates the development of small ventricles in at least 50% of patients who receive shunts in the first year of life (13, 16). Most of these children are shunt-dependent: when it malfunctions, signs and symptoms of increased intracranial pressure (ICP), combined with enlargement of the ventricular system shown by CT, make the diagnosis obvious. A shunt revison is curative.

The term "slit ventricle syndrome" (1, 2, 4, 6, 8, 18, 19) has been applied to a small subset of these shunt-dependent children who develop disabling chronic or recurring headaches associated with signs and symptoms of increased ICP and persistant small or slit-like ventricles shown by CT. The frequency of this syndrome ranges from 0.9% to 3.3% in children with shunts (1, 9, 10).

A variety of apparently contradictory pathogenic mechanisms have been described in the literature, including overdrainage of cerebrospinal fluid (CSF), periventricular fibrosis, intermittent proximal shunt malfunction, decreased intracranial compliance, and intracranial hypotension (1, 2, 6, 8–11, 18, 19). Much of the confusion regarding both pathogenesis and treatment has resulted from treating the slit ventricle syndrome as a single pathological entity rather than as a symptom complex with several etiologies. This chapter will discuss the various clinical manifestations of the slit ventricle syndrome and suggest the appropriate course of treatment for each.

DIAGNOSIS

It is essential to recognize that the slit ventricle syndrome is a constellation of signs and symptoms that may have multiple etiologies. The evaluation of the child with this syndrome must be systematic and comprehensive. Figure 7.1 summarizes diagnostic evaluation and therapeutic options.

For slit ventricle syndrome to be confirmed, the patient must describe headaches that are chronic, intermittent, and recurring. Information should be sought as to what precipitates, exacerbates, and relieves the headaches. Minor viral illnesses with their concommitant mild cerebral edema will often precipitate the headaches in a child with compromised ventricular size (20, 26). Patients whose headaches are exacerbated by activity and the upright position may be suffering from chronic intracranial hypotension (11, 12, 18, 19). Persistent cold sweats appear to be characteristic of intracranial hypotension (12). Whereas vomitting and severe headache are common, episodes of lethargy and obtundation occur less often but may herald a critical, life-threatening event (9).

Physical examination is often unrewarding, with the symptoms much more prominent than the signs. The shunt reservoir will commonly refill slowly after pumping as a result of the limited ventricular volume; however, when a shunt that previously refilled briskly becomes sluggish, a proximal obstruction should be considered. Head circumference should be measured: a relatively small (<50th percentile) thick calvarium is common. While papilledema is exceptional, fundoscopic examination may reveal diminished venous pulsations during symptomatic periods. A Parinaud's syndrome

79

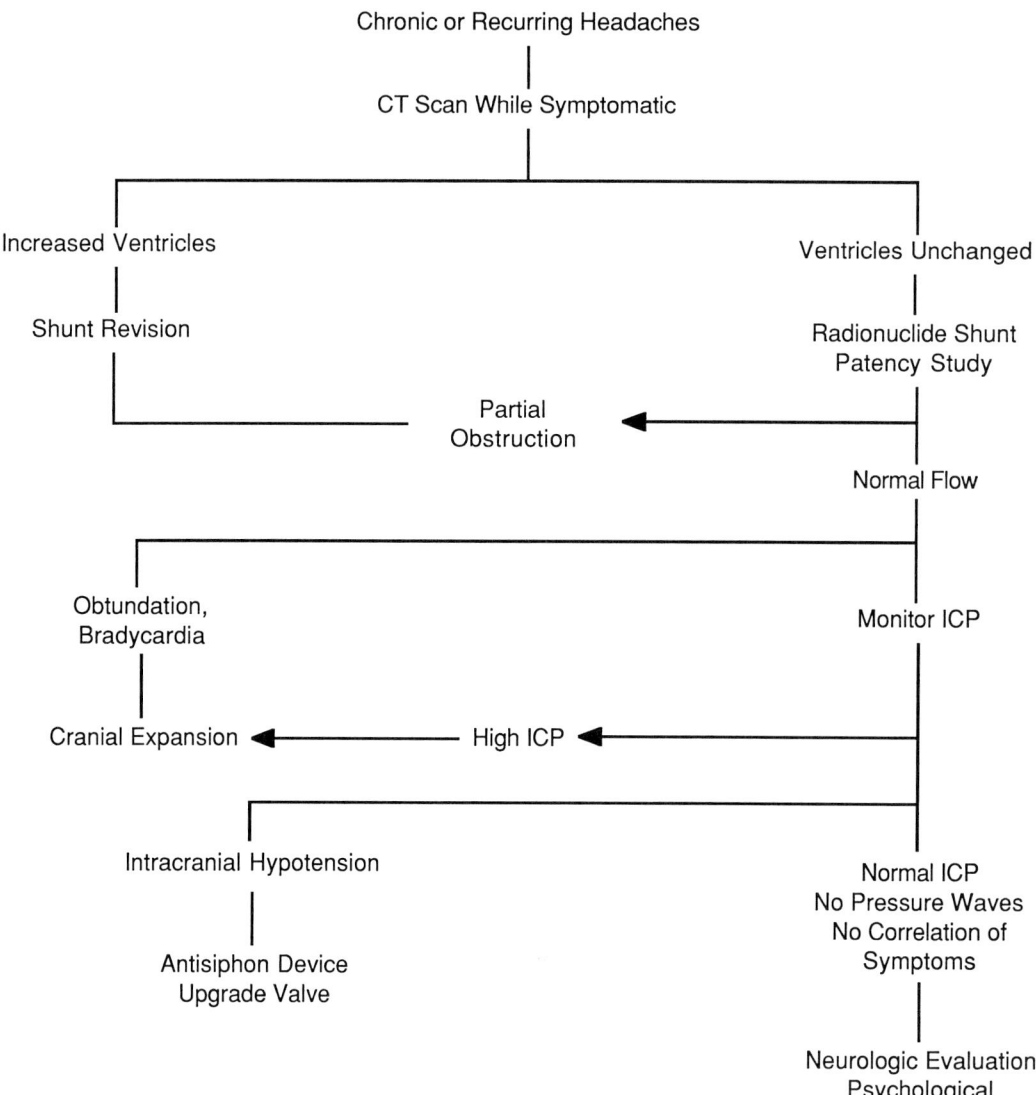

Figure 7.1. Diagnosis and management of slit ventricle syndrome.

may be seen with minimally dilated ventricles and should suggest shunt obstruction. Bradycardia, hypertension, and obtundation are ominous signs that demand prompt therapeutic intervention.

The CT scan is the paramount neurodiagnostic examination. It is essential that the study be performed during an episode of headache and compared to a baseline scan made when the patient was asymptomatic. Mild dilatation of previously slit ventricles may be the only objective sign of intermittent shunt obstruction (Fig. 7.2). Any increase in ventricle size requires an immediate shunt revision.

If the ventricles' size is unchanged, a radionuclide shunt patency evaluation is performed: partially occluded catheters will usually demonstrate a prolonged clearance time. Partially occluded ventricular catheters may provide adequate CSF drainage under routine circumstances, but may be unable to increase the rate of CSF drainage in response to increases in intracranial volume and precipitate the rises in ICP.

ICP monitoring is reserved for those children who have normal shunt patency evaluations as well as CT scans that are unchanged from baseline. We use the Camino system (Camino Lab-

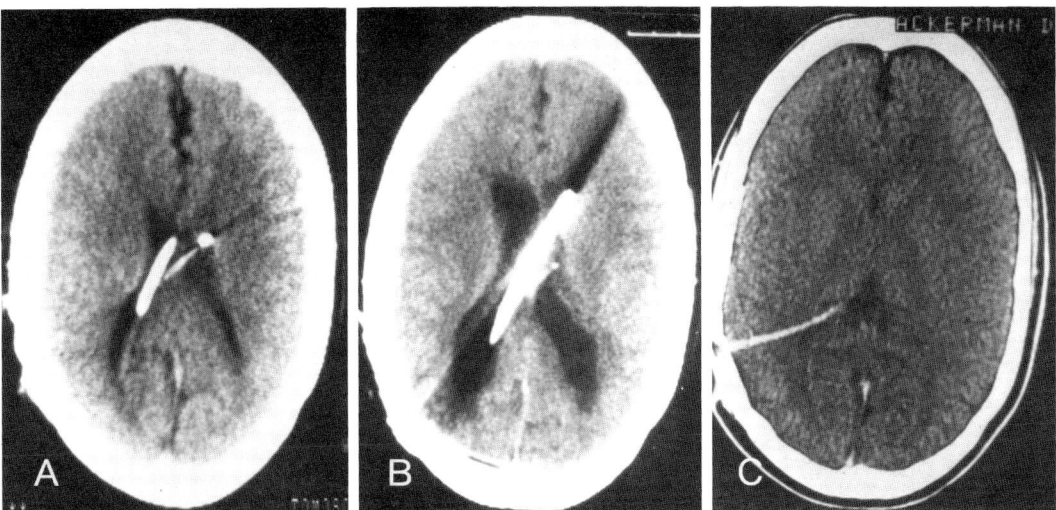

Figure 7.2. Case 1: A 13-year-old male with intermittent headaches, Parinaud's syndrome, and a malfunctioning proximal shunt. *A*) CT scan on admission shows small ventricles. *B*) CT scan 3 hours later discloses mild ventriculomegaly. *C*) CT scan following shunt revision demonstrates slit-like ventricles.

oratories, San Diego, CA) either through a modified subarachnoid screw or directly into the shunt reservoir. Patients are monitored for at least 24 hours, usually with a portable monitor that permits ambulation and simultaneous pressure recording with postural alterations. Paroxysms of increased ICP as well as symptomatic intracranial hypotension can be documented and correlated with the patient's symptoms through a concurrent bedside diary, which is kept by the parents or nursing staff.

TREATMENT

Since the slit ventricle syndrome can result from a variety of pathogenic mechanisms, therapeutic interventions must be appropriate for the individual's pathophysiology as determined by diagnostic evaluation (Fig. 7.1). Patients who present with relatively mild symptoms, a CT scan that is unchanged from baseline, and an associated systemic stress (such as a viral illness) may have a trial of medical therapy. A short course of corticosteroids and acetazolamide may significantly relieve the headache and return the patient to his premorbid state. If the clinical improvement is rapid (<24 hours) and the presentation relatively innocuous, no further intervention may be needed. If the child does not improve promptly or if the syndrome recurs within a few weeks, further evaluation and intervention is necessary.

Shunt revision is indicated in patients with increased ventricles or evidence of shunt malfunction on radionuclide shunt patency examination. The proximal catheter will usually be partially occluded with proteinaceous or gliotic debris. Since the ventricles remain relatively small, several technical points must be considered: *a*) The ventricles may be safely dilated by instillation of 10 cc to 15 cc saline over 30-60 seconds through the partially occluded ventricular catheter immediately before removal and replacement of the catheter; *b*) the old shunt tract should be used for placement of the new ventricular catheter. Attempts to cannulate the ventricle through a new trajectory are hazardous; *c*) when the proximal catheter cannot be removed or the new catheter cannot be reinserted through an old occipital shunt tract, a new frontal ventricular catheter insertion should be considered. Insertion of an antisiphon device may be performed at the same time.

About half of our patients have severe headaches with intermittent ICP elevations and normal shunt function. These children invariably have a relatively small (<50th percentile) head circumference and a thick calvarium for their age. In this situation we feel that cranial expansion is the preferred treatment, and carry out a craniotomy with morcellation of the posterior calvarium from the coronal suture to the inion as well as laterally to the squamosal suture (posterior calvari-otomy). Because there is often a deep midline keel indenting the sinuses that may compro-mise venous return, we believe that elevation and morcellation of bone overlying the sagit-tal sinus and torcular is essential. Although a subtemporal craniectomy can provide some element of cranial expansion with venting of pressure waves, we believe that posterior calvariotomy provides more skull expansion without any additional morbidity. We carry out the procedure on patients up through the teen years, and do not require the postopera-tive use of a helmet unless there are signifi-cant behavioral disturbances pre-operatively. Ten children have undergone the procedure thus far (July 1989) and in follow-up of up to 5 years there have been no long term compli-cations.

A small proportion of children will have a dramatic presentation of rapidly evolving ob-tundation, bradycardia, and hypertension with-out CT evidence of ventricular dilatation and with normal shunt patency. Cranial expansion will then provide immediate relief of the symp-toms of increased ICP. These patients will of-ten have persistent headaches that gradually re-solve over 6 to 10 weeks.

Treatment of symptomatic intracranial hypo-tension requires increasing the shunt system's resistence and eliminating the siphon effect. The simple addition of an antisiphon device to the existing shunt apparatus is usually curative. Occasionally, increasing the valve pressure may also be needed; however, upgrading the valve without addition of an antisiphon device is not advisable.

The intermittent occurrence of symptoms during school, work, or intensified activity may lead to misinterpretation of complaints as epileptic or hypochondriacal, resulting in in-appropriate referral to the school psycholo-gist, psychiatrist, or neurologist. The neuro-surgeon must document with serial CT scans no evidence of intermittently increased ventri-cles, obtain a normal shunt patency evalua-tion, and demonstrate a lack of correlation be-tween ICP monitoring and symptoms before considering the diagnosis of functional head-aches or seizures. Only after these studies have been performed and there is *no history of alterations in consciousness and vital signs* is psychiatric or neurological consultation ap-propriate.

Illustrative Cases

Case 1: A 13-year-old male had repair of a low lumbar meningomyelocele at birth fol-lowed by placement of a low pressure ven-triculoperitoneal shunt 1 week later. He pre-sented with 2 weeks of intermittent headaches and diplopia. Examination demonstrated a Parinaud's syndrome and sluggish refilling of a shunt that had previously pumped briskly. A CT scan (Fig. 7.2a) demonstrated small ventri-cles. Three hours after his initial scan, the pa-tient complained of increased headache and was noted to be obtunded. A repeat CT scan (Fig. 7.2b) demonstrated mild ventriculome-galy. At surgery the proximal shunt catheter was noted to be partially occluded. A new ven-tricular catheter and antisiphon device were in-serted. Postoperative CT demonstrated slit ven-tricles (Fig. 7.2c).

Comment: This patient demonstrates the im-portance of serial CT scans during symptomatic episodes to document shunt malfunction. Mini-mal ventriculomegaly in a child with slit ventri-cles is pathognomonic of shunt malfunction.

Case 2: An 8-year-old female received a shunt for aqueductal stenosis at 4 months of age. She required a single shunt revision 5 months later for a distal shunt malfunction. She was well until 2 weeks before admission when she complained of headaches associated with an upper respiratory illness. The headaches in-creased in frequency and intensity and she be-came obtunded on the day of admission. Exam-ination demonstrated a child arousable to pain, with a relatively small (at 25th percentile) cal-varium and a shunt that pumped easily and re-filled over 30 to 45 seconds. CT scan revealed slit-like ventricles (Fig. 7.3a) and a ra-dionuclide shunt study showed normal flow. ICP was measured at 300 mm H_2O after aspira-tion of all CSF. A posterior calvariotomy and morcellation were performed (Fig. 7.3b and 7.3c). Intraoperative ICP measurement demon-strated a fall to 10 mm to 20 mm H_2O follow-ing removal of the bone plates. The child re-turned to her premorbid state by the first post-operative day.

Discussion

Most hydrocephalic children, especially those shunted in the first year of life, will de-velop subnormal or slit-like ventricles. There is a small subgroup of these patients who will

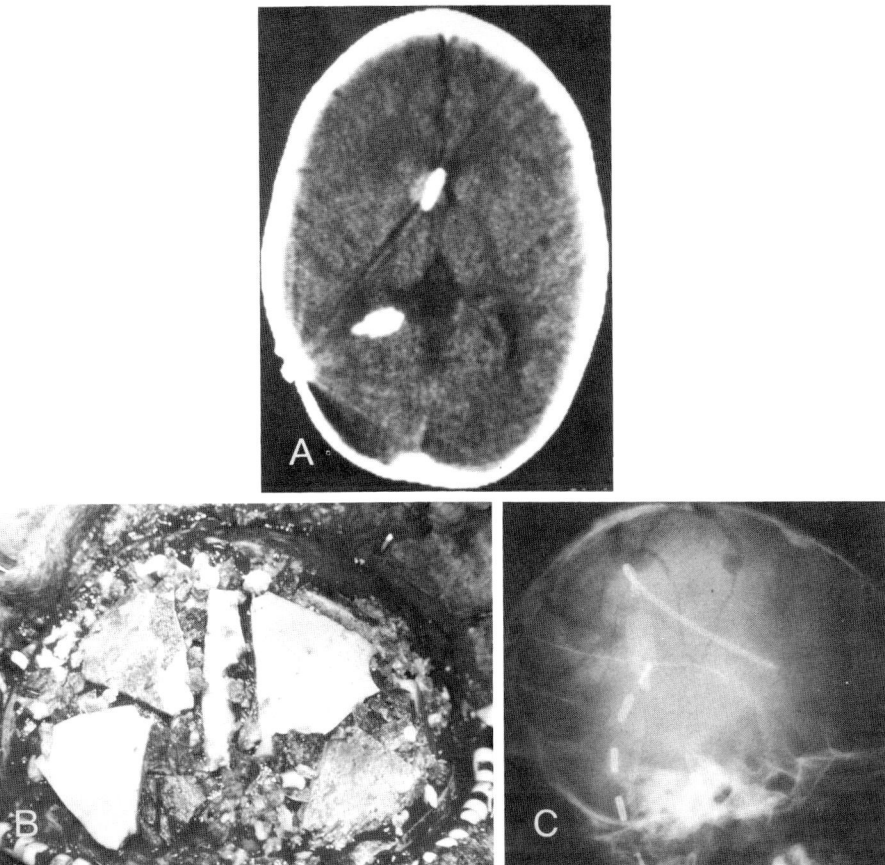

Figure 7.3.   Case 2: An 8-year-old female with progressive obtundation, slit-like ventricles, and normal shunt patency evaluation treated with cranial expansion. *A*) CT scan demonstrates slit-like ventricles. *B*) Operative photograph of posterior calvariotomy and morcellation. *C*) Postoperative skull x-ray.

demonstrate signs and symptoms indistinguishable from a classic shunt malfunction, but in whom ventricular volume remains near normal (5, 6, 8, 9, 12–14, 17, 18, 25, 26). Before the availability of CT scans, it was hypothesized that the chronic overdrainage in the upright position created a suction-induced collapse of the ventricular wall around the ventricular catheter, causing recurrent ICP elevations and, ultimately, complete shunt obstruction. This phenomenon has been noted in about half of the children with the slit ventricle syndrome seen in our institution: CT scans demonstrate transient increases in ventricular volume during episodes of severe headache.

Occasional patients with chronic shunt malfunction and patients with increased ICP may have severe headache as the only clinical manifestation (3). ICP monitoring and radionuclide shunt patency studies help to provide the cor-

rect diagnosis. The ventricles' failure to enlarge even minimally is enigmatic. The pathophysiology may be analogous to pseudotumor cerebri, with an increase in resistence to CSF outflow and altered intracranial compliance (secondary to increased brain stiffness from periventricular gliosis), permitting high pressures without ventricular dilatation (3).

Shunt revision has been curative in patients with intermittent obstruction of the ventricular catheter. Chronic suction-induced overdrainage in the upright position may contribute to proximal shunt obstruction secondary to entrapment of the catheter between collapsed ventricular walls (12, 14, 17, 24). We agree that altering the resistance of the shunt system with the simultaneous insertion of an antisiphon device when changing the ventricular catheter (9, 14, 17, 18, 24) is wise. This eliminates the suction phenomenon permitting slight enlargement of the ventricular system and 'freeing' of the trapped catheter. Unlike some authors, we do not routinely upgrade valve pressures (17, 18, 25, 26).

Several reports have suggested that small ventricles are in themselves pathological (10, 12–14, 17, 18, 24, 25) and have advocated elective upgrading of shunt valves to high pressure systems (25), high pressure systems with antisiphon devices (17, 18), or placement of an antisiphon device (12, 13, 14, 24) to prevent future complications. *We do not believe that this is a prudent therapeutic option.* The relative rarity of the slit ventricle syndrome in relation to the common occurrence of slit ventricles (1, 9, 10, 11, 13, 16) argues strongly against routine 'prophylactic' shunt revisions in the asymptomatic child. There is no evidence that a patient's long-term interests are better served by enlarging the ventricular volume. Such enlargement may result in symptomatic elevated ICP (21) and long-term cognative deterioration (7, 20).

Variations in shunt flow in the absence of demonstrable malfunction may contribute to clinical symptomatology. It is not necessary under most circumstances for a shunt tube to continuously drain at maximal capacity; however, in some patients a partially obstructed ventricular catheter may severely limit the ability to increase the CSF drainage rate in response to increases in intracranial volume, and thus precipitate the pressure wave. This would explain the observation that in some situations a proximal shunt revision is curative even with a normal preoperative shunt patency study.

Patients with patent shunts may demonstrate paroxysms of increased ICP. The pressure waves may evolve and dissipate rapidly. This most likely represents transient increases in intracranial volume secondary to increased cerebral blood volume (9). Whereas under normal conditions alterations in cerebral blood volume are buffered by an equal displacement of CSF from the ventricular system to the spinal subarachnoid space, this adaptive mechanism is lost when the ventricles are of subnormal volume and the calvarium is small.

Most patients with slit ventricle syndrome, with or without proximal shunt malfunction, do not develop life-threatening symptoms such as obtundation and bradycardia. In the small subgroup of patients who become critically ill, the head circumference is small and the calvarium

is thick. It is conceivable that early shunting of advanced hydrocephalus resulted in collapse of the cortical mantle and skull and subsequent craniostenosis (7, 9, 10). The treatment of choice in this situation is a cranial expansion, either by subtemporal craniectomy (5, 17, 26) or—preferably—posterior calvariectomy (9). These procedures provide an immediate bony decompression, acting as a "safety valve" to moderate rises in ICP. Additional relief is provided by calvariectomy through reduction in intracranial venous pressure (9, 15, 17, 22). It has been a uniform observation in our patients that the brain remains tense and engorged with blood until the bone overlying the posterior sagittal sinus and torcula is removed, when the brain becomes lax.

The symptoms of intracranial hypotension may mimic those of raised ICP: headache, nausea and vomiting, diplopia, paresis of upward gaze and strabismus, and lethargy (11). The history's pathognomonic feature is the onset or exacerbation of symptoms in the upright position (11, 12, 21). Bed rest, especially in the Trendelenburg position, provides dramatic symptom relief. ICP monitoring with documentation of negative pressures during symptomatic periods and no increase in ventricular size observed in serial CT scans is mandatory for this diagnosis. Failure to obtain the history of postural headaches and obtain ICP measurements can mislead the primary care physician to a diagnosis of an obstructed shunt: an unnecessary and potentially dangerous revision of the proximal catheter may ensue.

SUMMARY

The diagnosis and treatment of chronic headache in the shunt-dependent child and adolescent must be approached in a cautious, organized fashion. Revising a functioning shunt in a normotensive, small ventricle in a futile attempt to alleviate functional headaches may culminate in tragic morbidity and mortality. Careful planning must precede any contemplated surgical intervention. When intermittent shunt malfunction exists, accurate delination of the malfunction is essential to avoid several haphazard operations that can change a partial malfunction to total obstruction. Attention to the patient's history, serial and comparative CT scans, shunt patency examinations, and continuous ICP monitoring will direct clinical management and lead to the appropriate choice of medical, surgical, or psychiatric therapy.

REFERENCES

1. Carteri, A., Longatti, P.L., Gerosa, M., et al. Complications due to incongruous drainage of shunt operations. Adv. Neurosurg. *8:*199–203, 1980.
2. Collman, H., Mauersberger, W., and Mohr, G. Clinical Observations and CSF absorption studies in the slit ventricle syndrome. Adv. Neurosurg. *8:*183–186, 1980.
3. Dahlerup, B., Gjerris, F., Harmsen, A., et al. Severe headache as the only symptom of long-standing shunt dysfunction in hydrocephalic children with normal or slit ventricles revealed by computed tomography. Child's Nerv. Syst. *1:*49–52, 1985.
4. Engel, M., Carmel, P.W., and Chutorian, A.M. Increased intraventricular pressure without ventriculomegaly in children with shunt: "Normal volume" hydrocephalus. Neurosurgery *5:*549–552, 1979.
5. Epstein, F.J., Fleischer, A.S., Hochwald, G.M., et al. Subtemporal craniectomy for recurrent shunt obstruction secondary to small ventricles. J. Neurosurg. *41:*29–31, 1974.
6. Epstein, F., Marlin, A.E., and Wald, A. Chronic headaches in the shunt-dependent adolescent with nearly normal ventricular volume: Diagnosis and treatment. Neurosurgery *3:*351–355, 1979.
7. Epstein, F. How to keep shunts functioning, or "the impossible dream". Clin. Neurosurg. *32:*608–631, 1985.
8. Epstein, F. Increased intracranial pressure in hydrocephalic children with functioning shunts: A complication of shunt dependency. Concepts Pediatr. Neurosurg. *4:*119–130, 1983.
9. Epstein, F., Lapras, C., and Wisoff, J.H. "Slit ventricle syndrome": Etiology and treatment. Pediatr. Neurosci. *14:*5–10, 1988.
10. Faulhauer, K. and Schmitz, P. Overdrainage phenomena in shunt treated hydrocephalus. Acta Neurochir. (Wien) *45:*89–101, 1978.
11. Foltz, E.L. and Blanks, J.P. Symptomatic low intracranial pressure in shunted hydrocephalus. J. Neurosurg. *68:*401–408, 1988.
12. Gruber, R. The problem of chronic overdrainage of the ventriculoperitoneal shunt in congenital hydrocephalus. Z. Kinderchir. *31:*362–369, 1980.
13. Gruber, R. The relationship of ventricular shunt complications to the overdrainage syndrome: A follow-up study. Z. Kinderchir. *34:*346–352, 1981.
14. Gruber, R., Jenny, P., and Herzog, B. Experiences with the antisiphon device (ASD) in shunt therapy of pediatric hydrocephalus. J. Neurosurg. *61:*156–162, 1984.
15. Hakim, S., Venegas, J.G., and Burton, J.D. The physics of the cranial cavity, hydrocephalus and normal pressure hydrocephalus. Mechanical interpretation and mathematical model. Surg. Neurol. *5:*187–210, 1976.
16. Hirayama, A. Slit ventricle: A reluctant goal of ventriculoperitoneal shunt. Monogr. Neurol. Sci. *8:*108–111, 1982.
17. Holness, R.O., Hoffman, H.J., Hendrick, E.B. Subtemporal decompression for the slit ventricle syndrome after shunting in hydrocephalic children. Child's Brain *5:*137–144, 1979.
18. Hyde-Rowan, M.D., Rekate, H.L., Nulsen, F.E. Reexpansion of previously collapsed ventricles: The slit ventricle syndrome. J. Neurosurg. *56:*536–539, 1982.
19. Kierkens, R., Mortier, W., Pothmann, R., Bock, W.J., Seibert, H. The slit ventricle syndrome after shunting in hydrocephalic children. Neuropediatrics *13:*190–194, 1982.
20. Lorber, J., Pucholt, V. When is a shunt no longer necessary? An investigation of 300 patients with hydrocephalus and meningomyelocele: 11-22 year follow up. Z. Kinderchir. *34:*327–330, 1981.
21. McCullough, D.C. Symptomatic progressive ventriculomegaly in hydrocephalics with patent shunt and antisiphon devices. Neurosurgery *19:*617–621, 1986.
22. Norrell, H., Wilson, C., Howieson, J. Venous factors in infantile hydrocephalus. J. Neurosurg. *31:*561–569, 1969.
23. Nulsen, F.E., Spitz, E.B. Treatment of hydrocephalus by direct shunt from ventricle to jugular vein. Surg. Forum, *2:*239–403, 1952.
24. Portnoy, H.D., Schulte, R.R., Fox, J.L., Croissant, P.D., Tripp, L. Anti-siphon and reversible occlusion valves for shunting in hydrocephalus and preventing post-shunt subdural hematoma. J. Neurosurg. *38:*729–738, 1973.
25. Salmon, J.H. The collapsed ventricle: Management and prevention. Surg. Neurol. *9:*349–352, 1978.
26. Walsh, J.W., James H.E. Subtemporal craniectomy and elevation of shunt valve opening pressure in the management of small ventricle-induced cerebrospinal shunt dysfunction. Neurosurgery *10:*698–703, 1982.

CHAPTER 8

Shunt Infections

DAVID M. KLEIN, M.D.

INTRODUCTION

Infection remains a frequent and serious complication of cerebrospinal fluid (CSF) diversion. Mortality from shunt infection can range as high as 30% to 40% (18, 71), while survivors risk devastating functional loss from both spread of infection to the central nervous system and the interruption of CSF circulation. An important example is found in children with myelodysplasia, whose high prevalence of psychomotor retardation, previously attributed to intrinsic developmental abnormality, is found to result largely from shunt infection or chronic ventriculitis (30, 39, 64). Profound disability may also result from other secondary complications of infection, such as shunt obstruction, adhesive peritonitis, and septicemia.

EPIDEMIOLOGY

Although shunt infections have evoked a significant body of literature, the different results of prophylaxis and treatment leave many clinical uncertainties. The outcome appears to depend upon a number of variables that must be controlled to achieve consistent results. Some reports may be at odds because of differences in observed populations or reporting methods. In others, the specific location of an infection, its chronicity, the organism involved, and the host's shunt dependency may all be important in determining the success of a treatment program.

In 1970 Luthardt (34) noted an average infection rate of 13.5% among 17 authors. Rates ranged widely, from 7% to 29%, and it is not always clear whether these were for the population treated or the total number of procedures performed. Operative infection rates of 10% to 15% were common before 1980 (17), but the prevalence of shunt infection seems to be diminishing, both within individual clinics and as a general trend among reported series (18, 24, 59, 66). Currently a procedural infection rate of 2% to 5% is more commonly seen (10, 24, 29, 36, 43, 61, 66, 71). The specific reasons for this improvement remain unclear.

It can be estimated that 70% of shunt infections will manifest themselves within the first 2 months after surgery, with a steadily declining incidence of new cases discovered thereafter (18, 28, 44, 47, 59, 63). This clustering strongly suggests that most shunt infections are acquired at the time of surgery. Important determinants should therefore be discernable in the surgical techniques used, but unfortunately no such indicators have clearly emerged. Infection rates are substantially the same for ventriculoperitoneal (VP) and ventriculoatrial (VA) shunts, and for revisions as compared to primary placements (18, 25, 28, 50, 59, 63, 66, 71). Raimondi et al. (48) found the infection rate significantly lower for 1-piece as compared to 3-piece shunt systems, but one wonders if the absence of a reservoir in some one-piece shunts might not discourage CSF sampling in more subtle cases. Meticulous surgical technique, including reduction of operating time and tissue handling, the use of prophylactic antibiotics, and modern plastic adhesive barriers may be important elements in reducing these infections, but this remains statistically unproven. In analyzing 840 shunting procedures over 25 years George et al. (18) found that the surgeon's experience was the largest single factor in the prevalence of infections. Others, however, find no correlation of infection rate with the surgical team's composition, or with operating time, type of procedure, or shunt equipment used (50, 61, 63).

Younger infants and the very old are particularly susceptible (2, 18, 29, 47, 50). Infections at less than a year of age also appear to be more virulent, with a higher mortality rate (71). These factors suggest a lessened resistance for these age groups. The etiology of the hydrocephalus is also variously reported to be a determinant of infection rates. The author's total series of 422 includes an increased incidence among children undergoing radiation or chemotherapy for tumor, which could be a consequence of immunosuppression (29).

BACTERIOLOGY

Common skin commensals of low virulence, particularly *Staphylococcus epidermidis*, are responsible for most shunt infections. Approximately 10% to 20% of infections are due to gram-negative organisms and these are probably more common during the first 6 months of life (12, 42, 47, 50, 59, 61). The predominance of normal skin flora suggests that the shallowly placed shunt equipment may be easily contaminated from the patient's own skin. Bayston and Lari (4) performed preoperative skin and intraoperative wound cultures in the course of 100 shunt operations. Of these patients, 58% showed wound contamination by the end of the procedure, but only 55% of these contained organisms that had been present on the patient's skin before surgery. Shapiro et al. (61) compared the results of skin cultures from the operative sites in 413 pediatric shunt procedures to cultures obtained from 20 subsequent shunt infections among these patients. Only 4 (20%) showed organisms identical to those originally grown from the skin in the same case. The authors suggest that many shunt infections may occur as a result of contamination from the patient's nasopharynx, from operative personnel, or from the hospital environment. Such a conclusion, if correct, would militate against the effectiveness of systemic prophylactic antibiotics, which are presumed to work in part by reducing the patient's intrinsic skin flora.

PATHOPHYSIOLOGY

If most shunt infections probably result from direct contamination at the time of surgery, relatively few originate from other mechanisms such as hematogenous implantation, spread from contiguous tissues, or direct exposure of the shunt equipment.

A shunt may become contaminated by the fluid column passing through it, as from incidental meningitis above the shunt, or from perforated appendix with peritonitis below. Downstream distribution of contaminated CSF can result in the colonization of shunt equipment from an originating ventriculitis or in the delivery of infected fluid into the peritoneum, vena cava, or other absorption site. Secondary inflammatory changes, such as acute or chronic peritonitis, peritoneal pseudocyst formation, bacterial endocarditis, or bacteremia can follow. Obstruction of the shunt system is a common end result, either by clogging of its lumen with inflammatory debris or by inflammatory changes induced in tissues surrounding its distal point of discharge. The role of retrograde migration of organisms is disputed among studies done in vitro (5), but it has been clearly demonstrated clinically. Not only can tubing become involved, but organisms can migrate in retrograde fashion through a valve system to reach the ventricles or subarachnoid space (8, 52, 53). In general, therefore, it should be assumed that the entire shunt and its related tissues are infected if any part of the fluid column it delivers is infected, since local areas of sterility cannot be guaranteed from moment to moment.

Incidental blood-borne meningitis with secondary shunt involvement is usually more vulnerable to antibiotics alone, without shunt removal, than are infections developed by other routes, suggesting either a difference in the organisms' vulnerability to antibiotics or a reduced tendency for these particular organisms to colonize the shunt apparatus. *Hemophilus influenzae*, the meningococcus, and the gonococcus are notable in this respect (32, 33, 45, 46, 51), and the author has had similar experiences with pneumococcal meningitis.

Infection by direct implantation from transient bacteremia appears to be much rarer than might be expected, judging from the similarity between VA and V-P shunt infections, in their times of presentation after surgery and in the flora found. It is also important to recognize the difference between 'external shunt infection,' which may be viewed as an operative wound infection surrounding a foreign body, the shunt mechanism, and an 'internal infection,' involving the internal shunt surfaces and CSF column being delivered (43). External infections usually develop a more obvious and acute inflammatory reaction in the soft tissues surrounding the equipment, while internal infections can be more indolent in presentation. Internal and external infections most often seem to develop separately but they may coalesce later. Even the briefest direct exposure of the shunt, as by wound dehiscence or scalp erosion, is usually followed by infection, which is also initially of the external type.

The special characteristics of modern silastic shunt material and its interaction with bacteria are important in the pathophysiology of these unique infections and in the rational selection of a treatment plan. Staphylococci form discrete microcolonies on the surface of plastic prostheses, to which they adhere by secreting a mucopolysaccharide, the glycocalyx, that protects the colony and secures it firmly to even the smoothest surface. This phenomenon was noted in Holter shunts by Bayston and Penny in 1972, and has since been observed by others (3, 19, 20). Borges (7) studied the ability of human neutrophils and monocytes to adhere to shunt catheters and to phagocytose bacteria in vitro. He noted a failure of normal phagocytosis, apparently as a consequence of poor leucocyte adherence. Thus the shunt material itself may diminish the effectiveness of host defenses at the site of implantation. Guevara et al. (20) demonstrated different adherence to CSF shunts in vitro by different bacterial strains. They found that some bacteria remained attached within the shunts despite CSF flow at rates up to 200 times those normally seen in vivo. Using scanning electron micrographs, they also demonstrated surface irregularities in the walls of shunt catheters where bacterial microcolonies might be particularly able to survive despite treatment with antibiotics and irrigation. They believe these findings indicate that an infected shunt must be removed rather than sterilization attempted in situ. Infections diagnosed earlier, before they become imbedded in the fabric of the shunt equipment, should theoretically be easier to eradicate. This idea is supported by the clinical experience of Mates et al. (35). Of 48 patients with shunt infections, 8 were treated with only antibiotic therapy and 7 of these were cured; 6 of the 7 successfully treated patients were noted to have developed their infections within 2 weeks of shunt insertion or revision. It is unclear from this report why these 8 patients were originally selected for medical treatment only.

CLINICAL MANIFESTATIONS OF INFECTION

Presenting signs and symptoms of shunt infection vary widely. They may relate to inflammatory changes in contiguous tissues, to systemic consequences of infection, to shunt obstruction, or to a combination of these. Manifestations can be acute, but are often chronic and insidious. Among 267 infections involving both peritoneal and vascular shunts, Walters et al. (71) found frank meningeal or peritoneal signs each presenting in only 2% of the cases, while shunt malfunction and cutaneous abnormalities were each seen in 23% and fever alone presented in 18%. Cardiorespiratory symptoms presented in only 8 of the 50 cases of VA shunt infection (16%). Shunt malfunction and fever also dominate among symptoms reported by others (12, 42, 44, 59, 63). Although less frequent, anemia and failure to thrive are also observed. The classical syndrome of 'shunt nephritis' is produced by chronic indolent VA shunt infection with recurrent bouts of bacteremia, leading to an immune-mediated glomerulonephritis. The pathophysiology closely parallels that produced by subacute bacterial endocarditis (11, 14). The progression of renal damage can be stopped promptly by treating the infection and replacing the VA with a VP shunt.

DIAGNOSIS

Because signs and symptoms are usually nonspecific and because the consequences of the treatment itself can be severe, positive cultures are the diagnostic *sine qua non* in shunt infection. The physician must not only maintain a high index of suspicion, but he or she must be prepared to secure appropriate cultures, repeatedly if necessary, whenever the clinical picture is at all suggestive, and particularly in the presence of unexplained fever, shunt obstruction, or with any superficial swelling, tenderness, or erythema along the shunt's course. Such changes become highly suspect when they develop any time after the second postoperative day. Cultures taken during the course of any antibiotic therapy must be considered inconclusive if they produce no growth. Whenever possible, antibiotics should be stopped at least 72 hours before sampling. In suspicious circumstances, no shunt should be pronounced aseptic without multiple cultures, including anaerobic and fungal media, observed for at least 14 days. It is only by these means that the slower-growing, more easily suppressed anaerobes and skin commensals will be detected, and many times these organisms, often taken for culture contaminants, are the culprits in an indolent infection (12, 16, 49). At times a diagnosis can be confirmed only after several cultures are positive for the same organism. This underscores the need for access to the shunt CSF and suggests that a reservoir should be included in every shunt system.

In external shunt infections, cultures of wound drainage or subcutaneous aspirates from areas of erythema or swelling are usually positive. Care should be taken in these circumstances not to puncture the shunt mechanism at the same time. Where internal infection is suspected, the shunt should be punctured in an area free of cutaneous inflammation or abrasion, if at all possible. Meticulous preparation and technique should be used with every such aspiration, since the consequences of a false-positive culture can be far-reaching.

Schoenbaum et al. (59) have nicely demonstrated the reliability of cultures taken from different sources, in the presence of various types of shunts. As might be expected, blood cultures were more often positive (95%) in VA than in VP (20%) or ureteral shunt infections (0%). CSF removed by ventricular or lumbar puncture was a uniformly poor source of positive culture with any shunt type (7% to 26% positive). In shunts of all types, direct aspiration of shunt CSF accurately reflected the infection in 95% of cases. Thus aspiration of the shunt fluid column, the 'common pathway' of CSF diversions, would appear to be the best single external source of positive cultures in cases of internal shunt infection (41, 49, 59). The ultimate culture, that of the shunt equipment itself, produces a similar diagnostic return (92% to 100%). All equipment removed should be cultured, especially in the course of revision for apparently bland obstructive problems (15, 16, 71).

Unless immediate Gram stains are positive, microscopical examinations of aspirated CSF are otherwise only suggestive of infection at best. In shunt infections, aspirated CSF cell counts are usually only moderately elevated, in the average range of 50 to 200 cells per cubic millimeter. In fact, the cellularity induced in the CSF by the presence of the shunt itself may show little difference from that additionally generated by infection (44). Glucose and protein levels may be normal (16, 42, 44, 49).

TREATMENT

Although no single treatment strategy is universally accepted at the present time, the use of systemic antibiotics, usually with intraventricular supplementation, is generally agreed upon. The alternatives at issue are whether the shunt, as a contaminated foreign body, must be removed, and whether it should be replaced immediately or followed by a shunt-free interval with antibiotic therapy. Since each of these surgical maneuvers carries additional risks and tactical problems, the use of antibiotics alone—without interruption of shunt function—is attractive if it can be proven effective.

Immediate shunt replacement requires that surgery be undertaken in a sick patient, with tissues that may be inflamed and edematous if not still actually infected. Delayed replacement of VA shunts may result in loss of a useful vein, so that immediate replacement of this type of shunt has been particularly advocated (40, 42). Replacement of the ventricular catheter in a shunt-dependent, slit ventricle can be a hazard. Immediate VP shunt replacement may continue the discharge of inflammatory debris and antibiotics into the peritoneum as the treatment course is completed, increasing the likelihood of ongoing peritoneal scarring and further shunt obstruction. McLaurin and Frame (38) recently summarized their successful experience with 11 consecutive VP shunt infections treated by externalization of the peritoneal catheter and both intraventricular and systemic antibiotics. A new lower catheter was connected to the upper shunt system and reinserted into the peritoneum before completion of antibiotic treatment. This alternative is attractive in that it preserves ventricular drainage while temporarily eliminating peritoneal soiling or obstruction at the peritoneal shunt tip. However, partial shunt replacement has been reported elsewhere to carry an unacceptably high failure rate (16, 65).

Removal of the entire shunt with replacement after a period of antibiotic treatment usually requires interval external ventricular drainage (EVD) or serial ventricular punctures to relieve pressure, and these can be difficult to perform. EVD carries the potential for accidental disconnection of the tubing, superinfection, and significant extracorporeal CSF loss, but it becomes the tactic of choice if the infected shunt is also obstructed.

In 1961 Schimke et al. (57) proposed that indolent VA shunt infections could be cured by systemic antibiotics alone, but the results of this treatment have generally been unsatisfactory. Schoenbaum et al. (59) were able to clear only 5 of 30 VA and VP shunt infections by this means (16.7%); Shurtleff et al. (65) reported systemic treatment alone to be effective in only 2 of 39 VA shunt infections (9%). In each of these studies there was much greater success in cases treated from the outset with shunt removal as well as systemic antibiotics: 96% and 100%, respectively. None of these patients received intraventricular antibiotics.

It is now generally recognized that ventriculitis is a common accompaniment of shunt infection. To be adequate, antibiotic treatment must sterilize this ventricular pool as well as the CSF outflow column. Antibiotics administered systemically have frequently produced CSF levels that are inadequate to eliminate the organisms involved, particularly for penicillin-resistant staphylococci and gram-negative forms. The addition of direct intraventricular antibiotic instillations can raise CSF concentrations to consistently effective levels, and the combination of systemic and intraventricular antibiotics, selected according to bacterial sensitivities, improves the success rate of nonsurgical treatment (13, 27, 31, 54, 65, 70). In 1978, McLaurin (37) was able to report success in 29 out of 45 infections (64%) using systemic and intraventricular antibiotics, without surgery. However, others have not been so fortunate with this method. Yogev (73) collected data from 18 series, reporting their success rates with various treatment strategies. According to his tabulation, antibiotics alone have been successful in 36% of 195 cases. Antibiotics and immediate shunt replacement were 65% successful in 116 cases, and antibiotics with shunt removal and EVD or intermittent ventricular taps were 96% successful in 161 instances. A small, randomized study by James et al. (26) produced similar results: 3 of 10 patients were cured by intravenous and intraventricular antibiotics without surgery, 9 of 10 were cured with immediate shunt replacement and antibiot-

ics, and all 10 patients treated with shunt removal, EVD, and antibiotics were cured.

Most authors now recommend a course of antibiotics of 2 to 3 weeks duration in doses suitable for the treatment of meningitis, and the drug is specifically selected according to bacterial sensitivities. If possible, the same drug should be used for ventricular instillations, to produce a supplementary effect upon CSF drug concentrations. A single, daily intraventricular instillation is usually sufficient, depending upon the drug and the organism. Antibiotic concentrations in ventricular CSF can vary widely, however, because of differences in ventricular volume, transependymal flow, and the presence or absence of a functioning shunt or open aqueduct. Concentrations should therefore be checked at intervals. Trough levels, taken immediately before the next antibiotic dose is injected, are particularly helpful when compared to the concentrations known to be inhibitory or bacteriocidal for the organism involved (13, 27, 70). The continuous advice of an infectious disease specialist is indispensable in these cases.

The above figures clearly show that some shunt infections can be treated successfully with antibiotics alone. Unfortunately this group is not well characterized in the literature so that it is difficult to identify the patients who are most likely to succeed with this initial treatment strategy. The proper selection of an initial treatment is important: a succession of failed treatments can be expensive and crippling, if not lethal. In the series of Schoenbaum et al. (59), 6 of 43 patients died during their initial treatment of antibiotics only, while there were only 2 deaths among the 41 patients treated by shunt removal and antibiotics. Walters et al. (71) have shown that those given only medical treatment initially required, on average, more hospital days per infection (88 versus 71), more admissions per infection (3.2 versus 1.2), and suffered twice the mortality (36% versus 18%) as those initially treated with some form of shunt removal as well as antibiotics. Although it is unattractive at first glance, an immediate or delayed change in shunt equipment may in fact be a more conservative strategy in most cases, if the individual's clinical condition permits surgery. The striking difference in treatment results produced solely by the exchange of fresh for contaminated equipment persuasively supports the idea that colonized shunt fabric may often be impossible to sterilize with antibiotics, particularly when infection is long-standing and when staphylococcus is involved.

Several concepts that help in planning treatment seem to follow logically from the foregoing: a) When infection is demonstrated in any portion of a shunt system, the entire shunt usually becomes contaminated, along with the tissues at the ends of the CSF column, and these tissues also require consideration in the planning of treatment. b) The fabric of an infected shunt is frequently intractably colonized. Removal of this infected material can greatly facilitate a cure. c) CSF drainage and ventricular access must be maintained in most cases, if successful treatment is to be carried out. Table 8.1 shows the author's current treatment protocol as derived from these observations. It is admittedly a conservative strategy, shifting patients toward more stringent initial treatments than others might elect, but personal experience suggests this to be a small price for avoiding intractable or recurrent infections.

As soon as shunt infection is diagnosed, initial evaluation should include an x-ray series for shunt continuity and computed tomography (CT) for ventricular size and catheter tip position, if the patient's condition allows this. Broad-spectrum antibiotic coverage, in meningitic doses, is initiated as soon as routine blood count, serum biochemical profile, and blood cultures can be drawn. Assurance of adequate ventricular access and ventricular fluid drainage is an urgent concern. Old shunt equipment is removed and an EVD system is installed in the operating room according to the indications in Table 8.1. If the patient's condition does not permit this, simple exteriorization of the shunt tube can be performed in the treatment room, usually with minimum local anesthesia. This maneuver is insufficient, however, if the shunt system is obstructed between the ventricle and the point of exteriorization, and even when good outflow persists in this segment, the presence of a valve here may prohibit retrograde injection of antibiotics. A new EVD installation will be required, and intraventricular antibiotic coverage can then be initiated.

As soon as Gram stain and culture results are reported, specific antibiotics can be selected, with the advice and help of the infectious disease consultant. As indicated above, we have routinely used an antibiotic program consisting of at least 2 weeks of intravenous medication in meningitic doses, plus at least 2 weeks of intraventricular instillations. While the intravenous drug is dosed by weight in children, the intraventricular drugs are generally given in standardized increments that are adjusted according to trough antibiotic levels (13, 27, 70). An operative shunt change is preferably made after the infection has been under antibiotic treatment for 48 to 72 hours.

Whenever possible, a fresh operative site is used, usually contralateral to the infected equipment. The new aseptic shunt is installed first and after these incisions are closed and covered, the contralateral field is prepared, and the contaminated equipment is removed. If it is necessary to remove and replace a shunt in the same field, the author prefers to carry the preoperative antibiotic treatment for a longer period, perhaps 5 to 7 days. An EVD should be removed and a new shunt installed as soon as cultures of the external drainage become consistently sterile, in order to avoid superinfection. Ventricular fluid samples can become sterile with surprising speed—sometimes after only 24 to 48 hours—once the contaminated hardware is removed, but it is wise to wait for at least 3 sterile daily cultures before the new shunt is inserted, particularly since bacterial growth in these cultures may be supressed by ongoing antibiotic instillations. Ventricular fluid glucose levels and cell counts are not helpful in this respect (56). CSF cultures are taken to assess interval progress in all cases. The surgeon must be prepared to change treatment strategies promptly if there is any sign of therapeutic failure. Shunt cultures are also repeated starting 72 hours after the completion of all therapy. At least 3 daily cultures should be taken and each should be observed for a period ample to allow for the growth characteristics of the offending organism. For infected shunts originating in the spinal subarachnoid space, analogous access for CSF drainage and a similar program of treatment is established.

THE ACUTE ABDOMEN AND VP SHUNT SEPSIS

Special management is required for the VP shunt patient who develops signs and symptoms of peritoneal irritation, since these can be an expression of either covert shunt infection or of primary intraabdominal pathology, and each can lead to the other. Rush et al. (53) found 15

TABLE 8.1.
Shunt Infection Treatment Protocol

		Situation	Treatment
(A)	1.	Acute infections secondary to incidental meningitis (H. influenza, meningococcus, pneumococcus, gonococcus)	IV and intraventricular antibiotics only
	2.	Less than two weeks from originating surgery, without (C) characteristics	
(B)	1.	(A) Treatment failures	Antibiotics and shunt replacement
	2.	All others without (C) characteristics	
(C)	1.	(B) Treatment failures	Antibiotics, exteriorization or EVD, and delayed shunt replacement
	2.	Toxic patients	
	3.	Obstructed shunts	
	4.	Peritoneal signs	
	5.	Gram-negative intestinal organisms	
	6.	"External" infections	
	7.	Exposed shunts	

shunt-related abdominal complications among 300 children (5%) with VP shunts during a 10-year period, and an additional 2 VP shunt patients developed perforated appendicitis. In 13 of the 15 shunt-induced abdominal problems, there was descent of contaminated CSF from an infected shunt leading to the formation of ascites, pseudocysts, or abscesses. In 2 cases the shunt perforated a viscus and ascending shunt infection ensued. This can be a life-threatening event. Snow et al. (67) also, reported 2 cases of visceral perforation, and noted a 15% mortality among patients in 32 previously reported cases.

It is frequently stated that CSF withdrawn from the shunt in these circumstances will usually show gram-positive organisms in the case of a primary shunt infection and gram-negative enteric organisms when the infection is ascending from an abdominal origin. In fact, CSF removed from a shunt reservoir at the system's cranial end may be sterile when the problem is initially assessed, but this can be falsely reassuring, and one cannot afford to wait and risk the devastating consequences of gram-negative ventriculitis (60).

For these reasons and since a primarily-infected shunt that is contaminating the peritoneum will also require removal, the lower end of the VP shunt should be promptly exteriorized whenever clear-cut signs of peritoneal inflammation appear. The neurosurgeon and abdominal surgeon should consider the problem together. The peritoneal catheter can be easily exposed in its subcutaneous course; through a small transverse incision, a loop is elevated from below and the tubing is transsected. Cultures are taken from both sides, the upper end is connected into a sterile drainage system, and appropriate antibiotics are initiated. It is usually desirable to make a small injection of water-soluble contrast into the lower tubing before this is withdrawn in order to identify any visceral perforation or cyst formation. Such perforations generally do not require formal closure at laparotomy once the tubing has been removed. In the case of primary shunt infection, the removal of the tubing and its infected fluid stream can bring relief of peritoneal signs in a matter of hours. If laparotomy is required, this can then be conducted without further shunt contamination.

PROPHYLAXIS OF SHUNT INFECTIONS

The role of prophylactic antibiotics in shunt surgery remains undefined, but this certainly does not reflect a lack of interest. An abundance of papers has compared the prevalence of infection in patients undergoing shunt surgery with and without antibiotic coverage. A great variety of drugs and modes of administration have been used. Despite a plethora of reports, no single study has withstood scientific scrutiny sufficiently well to settle the matter, and there is no observable trend among acceptable reports.

Many earlier reports were anecdotal and without controls, or were reported as sequential trials with and without antibiotics (1, 29, 36, 55, 62, 69). The passage of time inherent in sequential trials can alter many of the variables considered to be important determinants of shunt infection rates, such as the operating team's experience, the patient population, and the observed general trend in infection rates over the years. The author's own report serves as an example (29). In this series 422 procedures were done using the same preoperative preparation and operative technique. An initial group of 93 patients received no antibiotic and sustained a 14.0% infection rate; the next 160 patients were given topical oxacillin and had a 5.0% infection rate; and the final 169 patients, who were given both topical and systemic oxacillin, had a 1.2% infection rate. No significant statistical difference was found between the control group and those given topical antibiotics, but those receiving both topical and systemic antibiotics showed a statistically significant reduction. Although the study was sequential, there was a sudden, stepwise decline in infection rate with each change in the antibiotic protocol, which argues against the significance of the author's growing surgical experience. However, other changes that might result from the passage of time are not well accounted for. This sort of study is not scientifically valid, but the results can still be persuasive in the absence of more solid data; the author continues to use prophylactic antibiotics, as described below.

Haines (21) has estimated that an infection rate of 0.8% to 5.7% is to be expected in clean neurosurgical cases. Tenney et al. (68) and Young and Lawner (74) have recently reported infection rates of 2.6% and 3.6% respectively for many neurosurgical operations performed without antibiotic prophylaxis. Shunt surgery might be expected to carry a slightly higher infection rate, because of the implantation of an avascular prosthesis, and indeed current infection rates for shunt surgery have generally fallen in the 2% to 5% range. As discussed above, this represents a general decrease in rates of infection reported over the past 20 years (24).

To demonstrate a statistically significant reduction from a 4% to 5% level by the addition of antibiotics requires a substantial series of patients. Tenney et al. (68) have addressed the specific problem and indicate that at least 1,600 operations would be required to confirm a 50% rate reduction from this level. If the antibiotic produced even less of an advantage, many more patients would be needed to demonstrate a difference. As many as 50,000 operations would be necessary to demonstrate a 10% improvement with antibiotics. None of the studies reported to date are large enough to achieve this short of significance, even though they may be well controlled in other respects. For example, Haines and Taylor (23) reported 5 infections among 39 patients (12.8%) in a placebo group and 2 infections among 39 patients

(5.7%) in a group treated with prophylactic methicillin, a reduction of more than 50% in infection rate, and they found "no statistically significant difference in infection or overall malfunction rate between the 2 groups." While this conclusion is correct, it could be the result of insufficient numbers rather than of ineffectiveness of the antibiotic.

The bacterial burden is an important variable that cannot be quantified in clinical situations and is therefore frequently not considered in studies of prophylaxis. Infection rates higher than the 2% to 5% ordinarily expected in clean neurosurgery, as suggested above, may reflect an unusually high level of contamination that could affect an antibiotic's effectiveness. For example, Younger et al. (75) report a sequential trial of single-dose intraventricular vancomycin for shunt surgery prophylaxis, in which there was a 14.1% infection rate in 127 control procedures, while a subsequent 103 patients given prophylaxis had an infection rate of 14.6%. The authors concluded that this mode of prophylaxis had no apparent benefit. It is not clear whether such results indicate that this antibiotic program is ineffective for shunt surgery in general, or whether it is only ineffective against a bacterial burden that is apparently higher than usual. Many other reports exemplify this (6, 58, 72).

In addition to other determinants of shunt infection, the specific antibiotic used, its dosage, and its mode of delivery are all critical considerations of assessing prophylaxis. Burke's study of guinea pigs (9) emphasized the critical importance of timing in the delivery of systemic prophylactic antibiotics. He reported maximum suppression of infection if administration preceded wound contamination or innoculation. Thereafter antibiotic effect diminished, so that when the agent was given 3 hours after contamination, it was totally without effect. This study suggests that in order to be effective, systemic prophylactic antibiotics should be started before the operation commences. Systemic antibiotics used in this way probably reduce population of skin flora as well as perfuse deeper tissues. Agents that are effective against typical shunt infection organisms may not penetrate CSF in effective concentrations after intravenous delivery, and others have therefore chosen to use topical or intraventricular antibiotics at the time of surgery. Again, reported results are inconclusive. From his review of topical antibiotic prophylaxis, Haines (22) suggests that procedures with intrinsically high risk of infection (greater than 15%) can be reduced substantially by topical antibiotics, but that there is no documented benefit for these agents in operations with an infection risk of 5% or less. Shunt implantation may represent a special circumstance, however.

In the absence of evidence to the contrary, the author has continued to use both systemic and topical antibiotics for prophylaxis in shunt surgery. For the past several years cephapirin, a second-generation cephalosporin, has been used both intravenously and topically. A dose for weight is given 6 hours before surgery when possible, and a second dose is given with anesthetic induction. During surgery a solution containing 2 mg of this agent per cubic centimeter of irrigant is used in wounds, shunt equipment is soaked in this solution before installation, and this solution (5 cc to 10 cc) is injected into the ventricle. Intravenous antibiotics are continued for approximately 12 hours postoperatively. The author's procedural infection rate continues at the 1.5% level.

The use of antibiotics constitutes but one form of prophylaxis. Meticulous technique must be maintained. Careful preoperative evaluation should ensure that shunt surgery is not conducted in an already contaminated field. For example, whenever possible, elective revisions can be delayed until shunt cultures are returned, surgery can be planned so as to exclude abraded skin from the field, and preoperative ventricular cultures can be obtained in infants with myelomeningocele, who might harbor a smouldering ventriculitis.

It has been the author's practice to recommend antibiotic prophylaxis for any patient with a CSF shunt who must undergo other elective surgery, who requires dental prophylaxis, or who has a serious respiratory infection. Antibiotics and dosage should be selected according to the organisms involved.

REFERENCES

1. Ajir, F., Levin, A.B., and Duff, T.A. Effect of prophylactic methicillin on cerebrospinal fluid shunt infections in children. Neurosurgery 9:6–8, 1981.
2. Ammirati, M. and Raimondi, A.J. Cerebrospinal fluid shunt infections in children. Child's Nerv. Syst. 3:106–109, 1987.
3. Bayston, R. and Penny, S.R. Excessive production of mucoid substance in staphylococcus SIIA: a possible factor in colonization of holter shunts. Dev. Med. Child Neurol. 14 (Supp. 27):25–28, 1972.
4. Bayston, R. and Lari, J. A study of the sources of infection in colonized shunts. Dev. Med. Child Neurol. 16 (Supp. 32): 16–22, 1974.
5. Bayston, R. Microbial colonization of cerebrospinal fluid shunts. Med. Lab. Sci. 38:259–267, 1981.
6. Blomstedt, G.C. Results of trimethoprim-sulfamethoxazole prophylaxis in ventriculostomy and shunting procedures. J. Neurosurg. 62:694–697, 1985.
7. Borges, L.F. Cerebrospinal fluid shunts interfere with host defenses. Neurosurgery 10:55–59, 1982.
8. Brook, I., Johnson, N., Overturf, G.D., et al. Mixed bacterial meningitis: a complication of ventriculo- and lumbo-peritoneal shunts. J. Neurosurg. 47:961–964, 1977.
9. Burke, J.F. The effective period of preventive antibiotic action in experimental incisions and dermal lesions. Surgery 50:161–168, 1961.
10. Chapman, P.H. and Borges, L.F. Shunt infections: prevention and treatment. Clin. Neurosurg. 32:652–664, 1984.
11. Dodd, H.J., Goldsmith, H.J., and Verbov, J.L. Necrotizing cutaneous vasculitis occurring as an early feature of 'shunt nephritis'. Clin. Exp. Dermatol. 10:284–287, 1985.
12. Everett, E.D., Eickhoff, T.C., and Simon, R.H. Cerebrospinal fluid shunt infections with anaerobic diptheroids (propionibacterium species). J. Neurosurg. 44:580–584, 1976.
13. Everett, E.D. and Strausbaugh, L.J. Antimicrobial agents and the central nervous system. Neurosurgery 6:691–714, 1980.
14. Finney, H.L. and Roberts, T.S. Nephritis secondary to chronic cerebrospinal fluid-vascular shunt infection: 'shunt nephritis'. Child's Brain 6:189–193, 1980.
15. Fokes, E.C. Jr. Occult infections of ventriculoatrial shunts. J. Neurosurg. 33:517–523, 1970.
16. Forward, K.R., Fewer, H.D., and Stiver, H.G. Cerebrospinal fluid shunt infections. J. Neurosurg. 59:389–394, 1983.
17. Gardner, P., Leipzig, T., and Phillips, P. Infections of central nervous system shunts. Med. Clin. North Am. 69:297–314, 1985.
18. George, R., Leibrock, L., and Epstein, M. Long-term analysis of cerebrospinal fluid shunt infections. A 25 year experience. J. Neurosurg. 51:804–811, 1979.
19. Gower, D.J., Gower, V.C., Richardson, S.H., et al. Reduced bacterial adherence to silicone plastic neurosurgical prosthesis. Pediatr. Neurosci. 12:127–133, 1985-86.
20. Guevara, J.A., Zuccaro, G., Trevisan, A., et al. Bacterial adhesion to cerebrospinal fluid shunts. J. Neurosurg. 67:438–445, 1987.
21. Haines, S.J. Systemic antibiotic prophylaxis in neurological surgery. Neurosurgery 6:355–361, 1980.
22. Haines, S.J. Topical antibiotic prophylaxis in neurosurgery. Neurosurgery 11:250–253, 1982.
23. Haines, S.J. and Taylor, F. Prophylactic methicillin for shunt operations: effects on incidence of shunt malfunction and infection. Child's Brain 9:10–22, 1982.
24. Haines, S.J. Antibiotic Prophylaxis in neurosurgery. Clin. Neurosurg. 33:633–642, 1985.

25. Ignelzi, R.J. and Kirsch, W.M. Follow-up analysis of ventriculoperitoneal and ventriculoatrial shunts for hydrocephalus. J. Neurosurg. *42*:679–682, 1975.

26. James, H.E., Walsh, J.W., Wilson, H.D., et al. Prospective randomized study of therapy in cerebrospinal fluid shunt infection. Neurosurgery *7*:459–463, 1980.

27. James, H.E., Wilson, H.D., Connor, J.D., et al. Intraventricular cerebrospinal fluid antibiotic concentrations in patients with intraventricular infections. Neurosurgery *10*:50–54, 1982.

28. Keucher, T.R. and Mealey, J. Jr. Long-term results after ventriculo-atrial and ventriculoperitoneal shunting for infantile hydrocephalus. J. Neurosurg. *50*:179–186, 1979.

29. Klein, D.M. Comparison of antibiotic methods in the prophylaxis of operative shunt infections. Concepts Pediatr. Neurosurg. *4*:131–141, 1983.

30. Laurence, K.M., Evans, R.C., Weeks, R.D., et al. The reliability of prediction of outcome in spina bifida. Dev. Med. Child Neurol. *18* (Suppl. 37):150–156, 1976.

31. Lee, E.L., Robinson, M.J., Thong, M.L., et al. Intraventricular chemotherapy in neonatal meningitis. J. Pediatr. *91*:991–995, 1977.

32. Leggiadro, R.J., Atluru, V.L., and Katz, S.P. Meningococcal meningitis associated with cerebrospinal fluid shunts. Pediatr. Infect. Dis. J. *3*:489–490, 1984.

33. Lerman, S.J. Haemophilus influenzae infections of cerebrospinal fluid shunts. Report of two cases,. J. Neurosurg. *54*:261–263, 1981.

34. Luthardt, T. Bacterial infections in ventriculo-auricular shunt systems. Dev. Med. Child Neurol. *12* (Supp. 22):105–109, 1970.

35. Mates, S., Glaser, J., and Shapiro, K. Treatment of cerebrospinal fluid shunt infections with medical therapy alone. Neurosurgery *11*:781–783, 1982.

36. McCullough, D.C., Kane, J.G., Presper, J.H., et al. Antibiotic prophylaxis in ventricular shunt surgery. I. Reduction of operative infection rates with methicillin. Child's Brain *7*:182–189, 1980.

37. McLaurin, R.L. Treatment of infected ventricular shunts. *Pediatric Neurological Surgery*, edited by Mark S. O'Brien, New York, Raven Press, 1978. pp 125–133.

38. McLaurin, R.L. and Frame, P.T. Treatment of infections of cerebrospinal fluid shunts. Rev. Infect. Dis. *9*:595–603 1987.

39. McLone, D.G., Czyzewski, D., Raimondi, A.J., et al. Central nervous system infections as a limiting factor in the intelligence of children with myelomeningocele. Pediatrics *70*:338–342, 1982.

40. Nicholas, J.L., Kamal, I.M., and Eckstein, H.B. Immediate shunt replacement in the treatment of bacterial colonization of holter valves. Dev. Med. Child. Neurol. *12* (Supp. 22): 110–113, 1970.

41. Noetzel, M.J. and Baker, R.P. Shunt fluid examination: risks and benefits in the evaluation of shunt malfunction and infection. J. Neurosurg. *61*:328–332, 1984.

42. Nulsen, F.E. and Becker, D.P. Control of hydrocephalus by valve-regulated shunt: infections and their prevention. Clin. Neurosurg. *14*:256–273, 1966.

43. O'Brien, M., Parent, A., and Davis, B. Management of ventricular shunt infections. Child's Brain *5*:305–309, 1979.

44. Odio, C., McCracken, G.H. Jr., and Nelson, J.D. CSF shunt infections in pediatrics. A seven-year experience. Am. J. Dis. Child *138*:1103–1108, 1984.

45. Petriarca, P.A. and Lauer, B.A. Ventriculoperitoneal shunt-associated infection due to haemophilus influenzae. Pediatrics *65*:1007–1009, 1980.

46. Petrak, R.M., Pottage, J.C. Jr., Harris, A.A., et al. Haemophilus influenzae meningitis in the presence of a cerebrospinal fluid shunt. Neurosurgery *18*:79–81, 1986.

47. Pui, C., Ch'ien, L.T., VanderZwagg, R. Shunt-associated bacterial infections in hydrocephalic children. Ala. J. Med. Sci. *18*:134–137, 1981.

48. Raimondi, A.J., Robinson, J.S., and Kuwamura, K. Complications of ventriculo-peritoneal shunting and a critical comparison of the three-piece and one-piece systems. Child's Brain *3*:321–342, 1977.

49. Rekate, H.L., Ruch, T., and Nulsen, F.E. Diphtheroid infections of cerebrospinal fluid shunts. J. Neurosurg. *52*:553–556, 1980.

50. Renier, D., Lacombe, J., Pierre-Kahn, A., et al. Factors causing acute shunt infection. Computer analysis of 1174 operations. J. Neurosurg. *61*:1072–1078, 1984.

51. Rennels, M.B. and Wald, E.R. Treatment of Haemophilus influenzae type b meningitis in children with cerebrospinal fluid shunts. J. Pediatr. *97*:424–426, 1980.

52. Rubin, R.C., Ghatak, N.R., and Visudhipan, P. Asymptomatic perforated viscus and gram-negative ventriculitis as a complication of valve regulated ventriculoperitoneal shunts. J. Neurosurg. *37*:616–618, 1972.

53. Rush, D.S., Walsh, J.W., Belin, R.P., et al. Ventricular sepsis and abdominally related complications in children with cerebrospinal fluid shunts. Surgery *97*:420–427, 1985.

54. Salmon, J.H. Ventriculitis complicating meningitis. Am. J. Dis. Child *124*:35–40, 1972.

55. Salmon, J.H. Adult hydrocephalus. Evaluation of shunt therapy in 80 patients. J. Neurosurg. *37*:423–428, 1972.

56. Scarff, T.B., Nelson, P.B., and Reigel, D.H. External drainage for ventricular infection following cerebrospinal fluid shunts. Child's Brain *4*:129–136, 1978.

57. Schimke, R.T., Black, P.H., Mark, V.H., et al. Indolent staphylococcus albus or aureus bacteremia after ventriculo-atriostomy: Role of foreign body in its initiation and perpetuation. N. Engl. J. Med. *264*:264–270, 1961.

58. Schmidt, K., Gjerris, F., Osgaard, O., et al. Antibiotic prophylaxis in cerebrospinal fluid shunting: a prospective randomized trial in 152 hydrocephalic patients. Neurosurgery *17*:1–5, 1985.

59. Schoenbaum, S.C., Gardner, P., and Shillito, J. Infections of cerebrospinal fluid shunts: epidemiology, clinical manifestations, and therapy. J. Infect. Dis. *131*:543–552, 1975.

60. Sells, C.J., Shurtleff, D.B., and Loeser, J.D. Gram-negative cerebrospinal fluid shunt-associated infections. Pediatrics *59*:614–618, 1977.

61. Shapiro, S., Bosz, J., Kleiman, M., *et al.* Origin of organisms infecting ventricular shunts. Neurosurgery *22*:868–872, 1988.

62. Shimoji, T., Sato, K., and Ishii, S. Measures taken to control shunt infections. Child's Brain *9*:370–371, 1982.

63. Shurtleff, D.B., Christie, D., and Foltz, E.L. Ventriculo-auriculostomy-associated infection. A 12-year study. J. Neurosurg. *35*:686–694, 1971.

64. Shurtleff, D.B., Foltz, E.L., and Loeser, J.D. Hydrocephalus: a definition of its progression and relationships. Am. J. Dis. Child *125*:688–693, 1973.

65. Shurtleff, D.B., Foltz, E.L., Weeks, R.D., *et al.* Therapy of staphylococcus epidermidis: infections associated with cerebrospinal fluid shunts. Pediatrics *53*:55–62, 1974,

66. Shurtleff, D.B., Stuntz, J.T., and Hayden, P.W. Experience with 1201 cerebrospinal fluid shunt procedures. Pediatr. Neurosci. *12*:49–57, 1985-86.

67. Snow, R.B., Lavyne, M.H., and Fraser, R.A.R. Colonic perforation by ventriculoperitoneal shunts. Surg. Neurol. *25*:173–177, 1986.

68. Tenney, J.H., Vlahov, D., Salcman, M., *et al.* Wide variation in risk of wound infection following clean neurosurgery. J. Neurosurg. *62*:243–247, 1985.

69. Venes, J.L. Control of shunt infection. Report of 150 consecutive cases. J. Neurosurg. *45*:311–314, 1976.

70. Wald, S.L. and McLaurin, R.L. Cerebrospinal fluid antibiotic levels during treatment of shunt infections. J. Neurosurg. *52*:41–46, 1980.

71. Walters, B.C., Hoffman, H.J., Hendrick, E.B., *et al.* Cerebrospinal fluid shunt infection. J. Neurosurg. *60*:1014–1021, 1984.

72. Wang, E.E.L., Prober, C.G., Hendrick, E.B., *et al.* Prophylactic sulfamethoxazole and trimethoprim in ventriculoperitoneal shunt surgery. J.A.M.A. *251*:1174–1177, 1984.

73. Yogev, R. Cerebrospinal fluid shunt infections: a personal view. Pediatr. Infect. Dis. J. *4*:113–118, 1985.

74. Young, R.F. and Lawner, P.M. Perioperative antibiotic prophylaxis for prevention of postoperative neurosurgical infections. J. Neurosurg. *66*:701–705, 1987.

75. Younger, J.J. and Simmons, J.C.H. Failure of single-dose intra-ventricular vancomycin for cerebrospinal fluid shunt surgery prophylaxis. Pediatr. Infect. Dis. J. *6*:212–213, 1987.

CHAPTER 9

Management of Hydrocephalus Detected in Utero

ROGER J. HUDGINS, M.D. and MICHAEL S.B. EDWARDS, M.D.

INTRODUCTION

The development of high resolution, real-time ultrasonography has allowed the accurate detection of ventriculomegaly in utero (24) and consequently has raised interest in the possibility of treating ventriculomegaly in utero. Because it is well established that the outcome of neonatal hydrocephalus is improved by shunting (16) it seemed obvious that the outcome might be further improved if fetuses could be treated before birth. Based on these assumptions, Birnholz and Frigoletto reported their initial experience with serial, percutaneous transabdominal drainage of cerebrospinal fluid (CSF) for the control of ventriculomegaly in fetuses (2). Clewell and others subsequently described the use of continuous CSF drainage by the ultrasound-guided, percutaneous transabdominal placement of ventriculo-amniotic shunts (5). The initial enthusiasm for prenatal treatment of ventriculomegaly waned after the publication of several reports documenting the frequent association of other severe, lethal abnormalities with ventriculomegaly, and the poor prognosis for survival and normal cognitive development in treated and untreated fetuses (3, 4, 6, 10, 19, 20, 22).

In this chapter we will discuss the diagnostic criteria for and evaluation of the fetus with ventriculomegaly, the natural history of this entity, the experimental and clinical methods that have been used to treat it, and the reasons why shunt placement in utero is generally not justified.

DIAGNOSIS AND IN UTERO EVALUATION

Recent improvements in the diagnosis of disease in fetuses and many subsequent advances in fetal surgery have been the result of the development of high-resolution grey scale, B-mode, real-time imaging and focused transducers for use in obstetrical ultrasonography (24). Improved visualization of anatomical detail has allowed greater understanding of the development of the central nervous system (CNS) and has allowed in utero diagnosis of pathologies such as ventriculomegaly (7, 8).

The fetal skull becomes discernable sonographically at 8 weeks. The intracranial space is largely occupied by fluid-filled cerebral vesicles that will become the lateral ventricles. Within these vesicles are the highly echogenic choroid plexi. The cerebral mantle is thin and difficult to distinguish because of its low echogenicity. At 15 weeks gestation the lateral ventricles are easily visualized and, except for the anterior horns, are filled with choroid plexus (Fig. 9.1); the occipital horns cannot be visualized at this time. By 20 weeks gestation, the lateral ventricles occupy a relatively smaller portion of the intracranial volume, but still remain filled by the choroid plexus. The slit-like third ventricle, thalamus, and temporal horns may be recognized. Also visible as a bright echo toward the posterior aspect of the midbrain between the cerebral peduncles is the aqueduct of Sylvius. The brain stem and basilar cisterns can be located by the presence of pulsating vascular structures within them. After 24 weeks of gestation, the ventricles become progressively smaller until they appear slit-like. Other than increased cortical convolutions, the brain undergoes little structural change.

Hydrocephalus may be detected as early as the latter part of the first trimester; in our experience, the earliest diagnosis was made at 13 weeks gestation. At this early stage hydrocephalus is characterized by a relative shrinkage of the choroid plexus in relation to the size of the ventricles (Fig. 9.2). Thus, as the ventricle enlarges it is no longer filled with echogenic choroid plexus. After 20 to 24 weeks gestation the choroid plexus is a less reliable indicator of ventricular enlargement, but by this time the ventricles are normally smaller than in the earlier stages, which makes abnormal dilatation more apparent.

The most frequently used measurement for detecting ventricular dilatation is the ratio of the distance from the lateral wall of the ventricle to the midline, to the hemispheric width (LVW/HW). This ratio, however, varies significantly depending upon the plane of section in which the sonogram is obtained and, because of the large standard deviation associated with this ratio, it is insensitive to an early appearance of enlarged ventricles. Fiske et al. (7) have described displacement of the medial wall of the frontal horn lateral ventricle toward the midline as a more sensitive measure of ventricular dilatation. This may be detected as early as 22 weeks gestation and occurs before the lateral ventricular wall is displaced from the midline, which changes the LVH/HW ratio.

If hydrocephalus is detected, a thorough ultrasonographic examination of the fetus should be performed to assess the possible presence of associated CNS and/or non-CNS abnormalities (e.g., spina bifida, encephalocele, Dandy-Walker malformation). An amniocentesis should be performed to determine the level of alpha-fetoprotein, which is elevated in the presence of an open neural tube defect, to search for abnormal chromosomes, and to determine the fetal sex (A male child with hydrocephalus may have x-linked aqueduct stenosis, relevant information for subsequent genetic counselling of the parents). Finally, maternal serum and amniotic fluid should be tested to rule out congenital infections such as rubella, toxoplasmosis, cytomegalovirus, and syphilis.

NATURAL HISTORY

Before treatment efficacy can be evaluated, the natural history of the disease process must be defined. Until recently, the prognosis for fetal ventriculomegaly has been extrapolated from experience with hydrocephalus in the newborn. This is obviously inaccurate because selection is biased toward infants who survive and may not include those fetuses with severe hydrocephalus and/or other severe systemic disorders. In several recent reports, attempts have been made to define the natural history of fetal ventriculomegaly (3, 4, 6, 10, 13, 19, 20, 22).

In 1984, Chervenak et al. (3) reported their experience with 50 fetuses with ventriculomegaly diagnosed by ultrasonograph: 60% had ventriculomegaly and associated abnormalities, 24% had associated spina bifida, and only 16% had isolated ventriculomegaly. Pregnancy termination was elected in 26% of cases, intrapartum death occurred in 14% (most of which were related to cephalocentesis), and 32% of patients died by age 7 months, most from associated abnormalities. Only 14 patients (28%) remained alive at the end of the study, 13 of whom required ventriculo-peritoneal shunting.

Of the 14 survivors, 6 had myelomeningoceles and 4 of these children had normal intelligence. Seven other children had associated abnormalities; only 1 child in this group had normal intelligence. The single survivor with no associated abnormalities had normal intelligence.

Ventriculo-amniotic shunts were inserted in 2 infants, 1 at 28 weeks and the other at 29 weeks of gestation. One shunt functioned for 4½ weeks, but the other shunt migrated into the ventricle. Both of these infants survived but neither is developmentally normal (microcephaly and hypertonia in 1; seizures, hypotonia, and hemiparesis in the other).

Serlo et al. reported their experience with 38 fetuses diagnosed with in utero ventriculomegaly (22). Five cases were detected early (<20 weeks) and pregnancy was terminated. Of the remaining fetuses, 23 were classified "severely affected" based upon ultrasonography. This group was defined by 1 or more of 5 criteria: *a*) multiple extracranial abnormalities; *b*) severe intracranial anomaly; *c*) severe fetal growth retardation; *d*) no recognizable cortex, even at the thalamic level; and *e*) retarded (microcephalic)

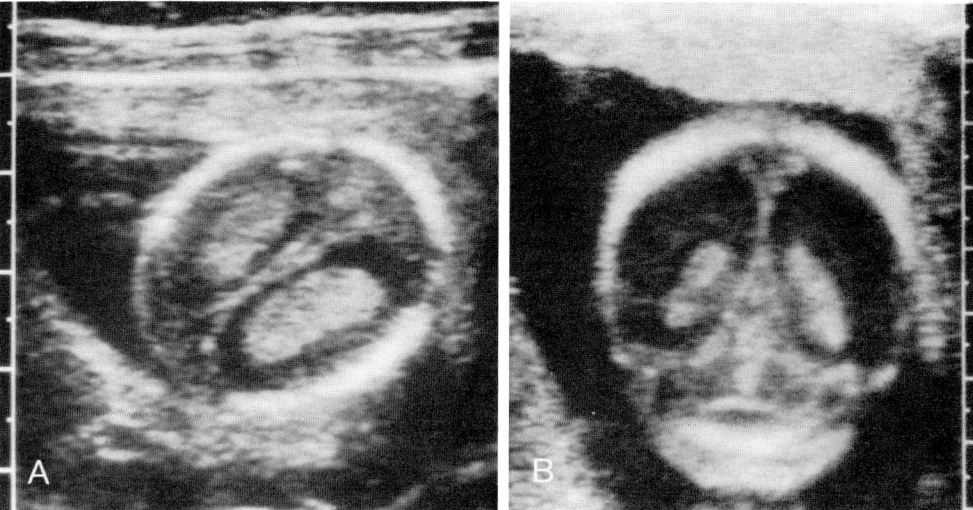

Figure 9.1.   *A*) Normal cranial ultrasound 15 weeks gestation. Choroid plexus fills lateral ventricles. Axial images. *B*) Twenty-one weeks gestation. Choroid plexus still fills ventricles, cortical mantle larger. Coronal image.

head growth. All these cases were treated without taking fetal considerations into account in planning obstetric care. Of the 23 severely affected fetuses, 19 died—2 in utero, 12 during vaginal delivery, and 5 during the first week of life. All fetuses that survived delivery had died

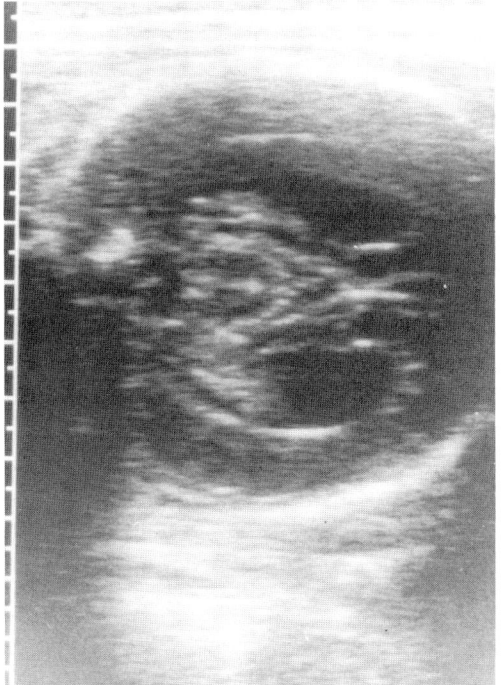

Figure 9.2.   Moderate fetal ventriculomegaly. Choroid plexus no longer fills enlarged ventricles.

by 9 months of age; 2 died after a shunt had been placed.

Ten fetuses did not have severe associated abnormalities. In this group, 6 have normal intelligence and 4 are severely retarded; 9 have required a ventriculoatrial shunt.

The experience from 4 Canadian universities was reported in 1985 by Cochrane et al. (6). The diagnosis of ventriculomegaly was made late in pregnancy in most cases; 32 of 41 cases were detected after 30 weeks gestation. Only 1 pregnancy was terminated and cephalocentesis for delivery was used in only 3 instances. The prognosis for a normal outcome was poor: 22% of fetuses were stillborn, 30% who were not treated died, 13% died after shunting, and 28% have developmental delay. Only 7% of the children are developmentally normal. Seventy-five percent of fetuses were found to have other CNS abnormalities in addition to ventriculomegaly. The authors noted that most of the fetuses in this series showed progressive ventricular dilatation with macrocephaly on sequential in utero ultrasonography.

Pretorius et al. reviewed 40 cases seen at the University of Colorado (20). Thirty-four (85%) fetuses died: 9 were aborted; 7 were delivered after cephalocentesis and none survived; 5 died of infection; 4 had multiple abnormalities that lead to death; 3 died in utero: 2 died of respiratory failure; and 4 died of unknown causes. Only 3 of 6 survivors were neurologically normal.

Recently, Nyberg et al. reported the experience from the University of Washington with 61 fetuses with ventriculomegaly (19): 84% had 1 or more major CNS or non-CNS abnormalities. Abnormalities of the CNS were correctly identified in 35 of 39 fetuses (90%). Of the 34 fetuses with non-CNS abnormalities, 27 had multiple abnormalities. There were 20 survivors (33%). They concluded that sonographic detection of extra-CNS malformations carries a poor prognosis and was associated with a uniformly fatal outcome.

We reviewed the outcome of 47 fetuses diagnosed with ventriculomegaly in utero over a five-year period by the Fetal Treatment Program at the University of California, San Francisco (13). In 20 cases the diagnosis was made early in pregnancy and was associated with other severe abnormalities. Pregnancy was terminated electively in 19 of 20 cases and none survived. In 5 cases, the diagnosis was made late in pregnancy and all fetuses had associated severe abnormalities. All were handled in a routine obstetric fashion and none survived. Of the remaining 22 fetuses, 19 had stable and 2 had progressive ventriculomegaly; in 1 case ventriculomegaly resolved in utero. Of these 22 fetuses, 19 have survived; 13 children have normal intellectual development and 6 are moderately to severely delayed. Associated abnormalities were detected by in utero ultrasonography in 74% of cases, but there was a false-negative detection rate of 20%. Outcome was not related to the degree of ventriculomegaly; intellectual development was normal in 2 infants born with severe ventriculomegaly and most mentally deficient infants had only moderately enlarged ventricles.

We also found that fetuses theoretically most likely to benefit from intervention, those with progressive, isolated ventriculomegaly, were not encountered frequently. In our series, only 2 of 47 fetuses fit this criterion. Both were treated by term delivery and ex utero shunting and are neurologically normal.

We have compiled the data from these series (excluding the study of Nyberg et al. [19], which is not strictly a pre-partum evaluation) and of 280 cases of fetal ventriculomegaly, only 74 fetuses survived. The most frequent cause of death was iatrogenic (pregnancy termination, cephalocentesis), but the mortality rate is high even without such intervention. Among the 63 survivors in whom outcome was

assessed only 31 (49%) had normal intelligence and the remaining children were moderately to severely retarded. This poor outcome is largely related to the high prevalence of associated abnormalities: 81% of the total of 280 fetuses had associated abnormalities, not all of which were detected by in utero ultrasonography; the false-negative rate was between 20% and 39%.

Thus it seems clear that the prognosis for the fetus with ventriculomegaly is poor: there is a 70% mortality rate and only 50% of survivors will have normal intellectual development. Even in the hands of experienced ultrasonographers, severe associated abnormalities may not be detected. In addition, the fetus most likely to benefit from in utero shunting (progressive, isolated ventriculomegaly) is rarely encountered and, in our experience, may be managed appropriately by term delivery and ex utero shunting.

EXPERIMENTAL MODELS

The difficulties in developing and maintaining an animal model of fetal hydrocephalus and the technical problems inherent in placing a functioning shunt in utero have precluded satisfactory laboratory studies of the efficacy of in utero shunting. The first experimental study was performed by Michejda and Hodgen in 1981 (17). They reported the development and use of the hydrocephalic antenatal vent for intrauterine treatment (HAVIT) for the treatment of fetal hydrocephalus produced in rhesus monkeys.

The HAVIT is a stainless steel device that has a ball-and-spring flow valve set to allow CSF drainage into the amniotic fluid when the intracranial pressure (ICP) exceeds 60 mm water. It was placed via hysterotomy performed in the late second or early trimester when the cranial bones of the monkey fetus are sufficiently ossified to allow the device to be anchored into the skull. Hydrocephalus was produced in the fetus by intramuscular injection of triamcinolone acetonide (10 mg/kg) in the gravid monkey on Days 21, 23, and 25 of pregnancy. Hydrocephalus was confirmed by plain x-ray films, ultrasonography, and fetoscopy. At Days 115 to 125 of pregnancy, a hysterotomy was performed and ICP was monitored by a pressure monitor inserted into the fetus' lateral ventricle. The intraventricular pressure in control monkeys was in the range of 45 to 55 mm water, but was consistently greater than 100 mm water in hydrocephalic fetuses.

While their results were not tabulated, Michejda and Hodgen (17) state that most of the untreated hydrocephalic fetuses manifested intrauterine growth retardation, confirmed severe hydrocephalus, frequent seizures, progressive motor weakness, and frequently died 10 to 14 days after delivery. In contrast, most of the treated monkeys showed progressive physical dexterity, grew at near-normal rates, and did not die. They concluded that fetal hydrocephalus could be diagnosed and treated in utero.

In the only other major experimental study of in utero treatment of hydrocephalus, we produced hydrocephalus in fetal lambs and rhesus monkeys by injecting kaolin through the surgically-exposed uterine wall into the cisterna magna of the fetus (11). At approximately 20 days after the kaolin injection, fetuses were exposed by hysterotomy and 1 of 3 different shunting procedures was performed: ventriculo-amniotic, ventriculo-right atrial, or ventriculopleural. A standard multiholed ventricular catheter and a distal catheter with a one-way, lower-pressure slit valve was used. Delivery was performed at term by cesarean section, viability was determined 2 hours after birth, and animals were sacrificed and both gross and microscopic examinations of the brain were performed.

Unshunted lambs had enlarged heads, bulging fontanels, and marked ventriculomegaly in all instances. The inflammatory infiltrate caused by the kaolin was found in the leptomeninges around the brain stem and cerebellum, and occasionally extended into the fourth ventricle and aqueduct of Sylvius. In contrast, most shunted fetal lambs had a more normal head size, overriding sutures, preservation of the anatomy of the cerebral hemispheres, and ventricles of normal size. Viability was also significantly greater for shunted (70%) than for unshunted (14%) fetuses. In shunted animals, the kaolin-induced inflammatory response extended onto the ependymal lining of the lateral ventricles and the ventricle was often obliterated by dense adhesions. This was felt to be caused by ventricular reflux of the kaolin secondary to reversal of CSF flow after shunting. Shunting did not significantly alter the histopathology in rhesus monkeys, probably because of a high incidence of shunt malfunction. Complications of the procedure included subdural hematomas and hygromas, shunt infection, and improper shunt tip placement that was seen in both groups of animals.

The results of experimental studies in animals show that in utero shunting improves overall survival and reduces ventriculomegaly. However, significant complications were associated with the procedure. We feel that the pathophysiology of fetal hydrocephalus and the shunting technique should be explored more vigorously in animal models before the technique is used to treat human fetuses.

CLINICAL EXPERIENCE

Early experience with CSF drainage in utero from hydrocephalic fetuses was gained during attempts to reduce the size of the fetuses' head in order to effect safe vaginal delivery, and not for the treatment of ventriculomegaly per se. In 1966, Barke et al. reported the first case of fetal ventriculomegaly confirmed by plain x-ray films (1). An air ventriculogram was obtained by transcervical placement of an 18-gauge spinal needle into the ventricle in a term infant. The day after the ventriculogram was obtained, the child was delivered stillborn. Nitrous oxide and iodine-based contrast agents have also been used to visualize fetal ventriculomegaly (18, 21).

Kellner et al. reported documenting ventriculomegaly in a 36-week-old fetus by performing a transabdominal, ultrasonically guided air ventriculogram (14). Because an L/S ratio of 1.69 had been found from the results of a previous amniocentesis, it had been decided that delivery should not be attempted, and that if it could be documented that cortical damage was not severe, a valve-regulated ventriculo-amniotic shunt would be placed. The ventriculogram showed an absence of cortex in the parietal and occipital regions, and it was felt that the fetus was not a good candidate for in utero shunting. After transvaginal cephalocentesis, the fetus was delivered stillborn at 39 weeks and was found at autopsy to have multiple abnormalities.

In 1981, Birnholz and Frigoletto reported the use of serial percutaneous cephalocentesis to treat hydrocephalus in utero (2). The diagnosis of hydrocephalus was made at 24 weeks in what was felt to be an otherwise normal fetus. With ultrasound guidance, serial percutaneous cephalocentesis was performed beginning at 25 weeks and continued at 1 to 2 week intervals until the infant was delivered by cesarian section at 34 weeks. Postnatally, a CT scan revealed asymmetric hydrocephalus, a posterior midline cyst, and absence of the corpus callosum. A ventriculo-peritoneal shunt was placed. The child was subsequently found to have Becker's muscular dystrophy and a seizure disorder and remains developmentally retarded.

Serial cephalocentesis requires multiple cerebral punctures and does not allow consistent reduction of elevated ICP. The first instances of continuous drainage of CSF to treat hydrocephalus in utero were reported by Clewell et al. (5) and subsequently by Frigoletto et al. (9) in 1982. Clewell et al. reported the insertion of a ventriculo-amniotic shunt in a 23-week-old male fetus; there was a family history of X-linked aqueductal stenosis, but no other abnormalities were detected on ultrasonograms. They used a silastic shunt with a unidirectional, flow-limiting valve that was placed transabdominally with ultrasound guidance through the posterior parietal skull and brain into the lateral ventricle. After shunt insertion, serial ultrasonograms showed a decrease in size of the ventricles, the LVW/HW ratio, and the biparietal diameter, as well as an increase in the thickness of the cortical mantle. An increase in the ventricles' size that was seen between 32 and 34 weeks gestation suggested that the shunt had malfunctioned, and the infant was delivered by cesarean section. Postpartum examination showed that the shunt catheter was occluded by tissue that had grown into the lumen and valve. A ventriculoperitoneal shunt was placed. At the last follow-up (52 weeks gestational age), the infant had poor head control, contractures of the hands, and did follow objects, but had developed a social smile.

Frigoletto et al. placed a ventriculo-amniotic shunt in a 23-week-old fetus whose only other known abnormality was a facial cleft. The initial attempt was unsuccessful. CSF was withdrawn with a 13-gauge needle, and the catheter jammed in the needle during an attempt to insert it into the ventricle. The catheter was lost in the peritoneal cavity when the needle was withdrawn from the fetus. A second catheter was then placed with difficulty. Subsequent serial ultrasonograms showed a slight but progressive increase in the size of the ventricles. Therefore, a valveless piece of silastic tubing

was placed into the ventricle and a progressive decrease in the size of the ventricles was seen on serial ultrasonograms. The infant was delivered by cesarean section at 28 weeks because of transcervical leakage of amniotic fluid; at delivery, CSF was dripping freely from the valveless silastic tube but not from the valved catheter. A ventriculoperitoneal shunt was placed at 2 weeks of age. The patient's course was complicated by diabetes insipidus, seizures, and possibly by sepsis; he died of cardiac arrest at 5½ weeks of age. It was speculated that amniotic fluid had refluxed into the venticular system through the valveless catheter, which might produce aseptic meningitis. A CSF cell count was not reported and an autopsy was not performed.

Because of the increasing interest in the in utero treatment of fetal disorders, in 1982 the Kroc Foundation sponsored a conference for workers involved in fetal treatment (12). The available experimental and clinical research on the treatment of fetuses, including the treatment of fetal hydrocephalus, was reviewed. At the time of conference 8 fetuses had been treated by in utero ventriculo-amniotic shunting. A decrease in ventricular size was seen in 7 fetuses and shunt dislodgment required revision in 3 fetuses. Six survived and required ventriculo-peritoneal shunts after delivery. Efficacy could not be determined without long-term follow-up, and participants elected to establish a registry of treated cases to allow evaluation of the "benefits and liabilities" of fetal surgery. The most promising candidate for in utero shunting was considered to be the fetus with progressive ventriculomegaly who was too immature for delivery and placement of a shunt postnatally, had a normal karyotype, and had no other severe abnormalities identified on ultrasonograms.

Even as enthusiasm for in utero shunting grew, many experts called for restraint. Several theoretical concerns were raised by Venes in 1983 (23), including the paucity of evidence for a correlation between the size of the ventricle and eventual psychomotor development. Because CSF flow may be necessary for the development of CSF pathways, concern was raised that diversion of CSF by in utero shunting too early in gestation could cause reversible hydrocephalus to become irreversible. Moreover, Venes argued that placement of in utero shunts was not justified until the natural history of fetal hydrocephalus had been defined. She suggested that in utero shunting of human fetuses be halted until these questions had been answered.

These concerns so dampened the initial enthusiasm for in utero shunting that the International Fetal Surgery Registry, which included 29 centers in 7 countries, recorded only 41 attempts at in utero ventricular drainage between 1982 and 1985 (15). This series represents the largest compilation of fetuses treated for hydrocephalus. Of 41 fetuses, 39 were treated by ventriculo-amniotic shunting and 2 by serial ventricular punctures. In most instances, a silastic shunt with a one-way valve was used. The mean gestational age at diagnosis was 25 weeks, and the mean gestational age at treatment was 27 weeks.

Seven of the fetuses died (17%), 1 before and 6 after birth. The stillborn fetus died as the result of needle trauma to the brain stem at the time of ventriculo-amniotic shunt placement. Three of the 6 postpartum deaths resulted from premature labor presumed secondary to chorioamnionitis from shunt placement. Thus, the procedure-related mortality rate was 10%.

The 34 surviving infants were followed for an average of 8.2 months. Twelve infants, all with aqueductal stenosis, were normal (35%); 22 have various degrees of neurological and systemic deficits. Four are mildly to moderately handicapped (12%), while 18 were classified as having severe deficits and gross developmental delay (53%). Other significant non-CNS abnormalities were found in 22% of infants. It appeared that fetuses with aqueductal stenosis received the most benefit from in utero shunting, but when this group was compared with fetuses with aqueductal stenosis treated after delivery, it was found that fetal intervention improved survival without functional outcome.

RECOMMENDED MANAGEMENT

The etiology of fetal hydrocephalus is variable and the pathogenesis and natural history are not fully defined. Before improved shunting systems and techniques will be of benefit, it will be necessary to have a better understanding of the effects of these variables and to have improved methods for the in utero diagnosis of other abnormalities associated with ventricular enlargement. Despite these limitations, we have formulated the following approach to

treatment based on the best information currently available (Fig. 9.3).

After the diagnosis of fetal ventriculomegaly has been made, a high-resolution ultrasonogram screening examination should be performed to identify any associated abnormalities. An amniocentesis should be performed to determine the presence or absence of chromosomal abnormalities, rubella, cytomegalovirus, and alphafetoprotein and acetylcholinesterase levels. Aggressive treatment may not be appropriate if ventriculomegaly is severe, if there are significant associated abnormalities, or if there is evidence of intrauterine infection. In the absence of these factors, fetuses are followed by weekly sonograms and, if the size of the ventricles remains stable, the fetus is followed to term. If there is cephalopelvic disproportion at term, cesarean section is preferred. After birth, the neonate is evaluated clinically and by ultrasonography, CT scanning, or magnetic resonance imaging and a decision on treatment is made. If hydrocephalus is not confirmed at the initial evaluation, the patient is followed clinically and by serial ultrasonography for signs of hydrocephalus that may develop many months after delivery. Should hydrocephalus occur, a shunting procedure is performed.

If progressive ventriculomegaly is documented by serial ultrasonography, the choice of treatment depends upon gestational age and an assessment of fetal viability. In a fetus older than 32 weeks gestation, preterm cesarean section is performed and a shunt is placed postnatally. For fetuses less than 32 weeks of gestational age, the risk of pulmonary immaturity must be weighed against the potential damage that may be caused by progressive ventriculomegaly. At present, we feel there is no evidence to justify placement of a shunt in utero.

Management should be based upon the parents' decision after consultation with physicians familiar with congenital neurologic disorders. Parents should be informed of the current knowledge of the natural history of fetal hydrocephalus, the possible etiology of hydrocephalus in their particular case, the presence or absence of associated abnormalities, and the therapeutic alternatives, including termination of pregnancy for a previable fetus. The extremely stressful nature of this situation must be understood and emotional support from social workers and/or clergy should be made available to the family.

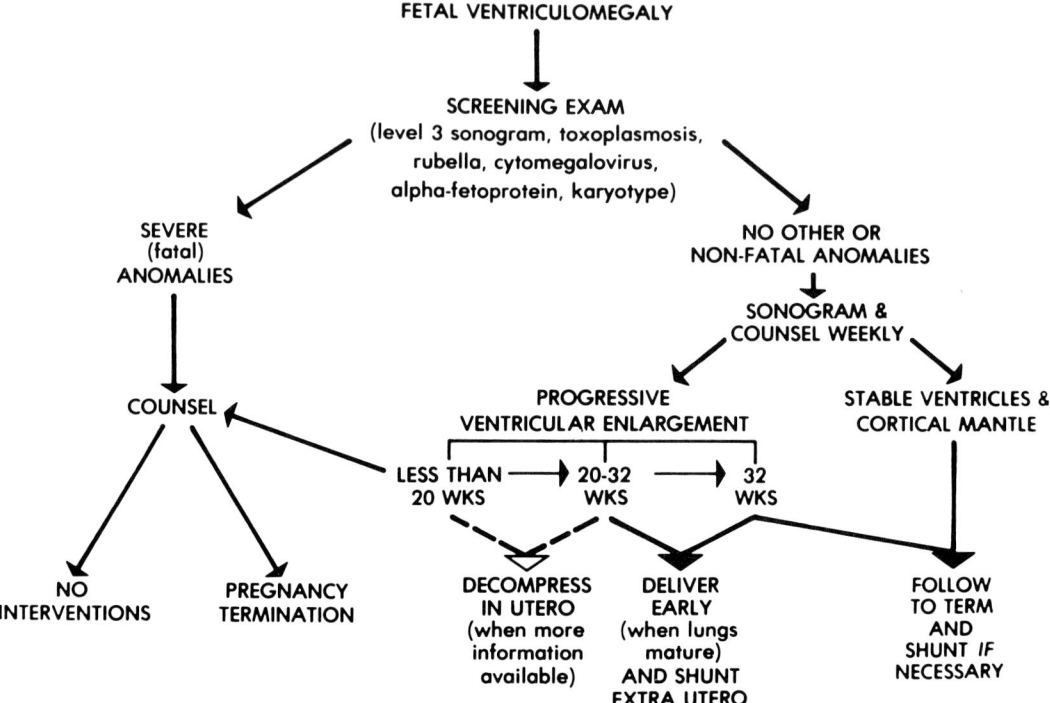

Figure 9.3. Suggested scheme for evaluation and treatment of fetal ventriculomegaly. (Used with permission from Edwards MSB, *Clin Neurosurg, 33:*347–357, 1986.)

REFERENCES

1. Barke, M.W., Scarbough, J.L., and O'Gorman, L. Intrauterine ventriculography of the hydrocephalic fetus. Obstet. Gynecol. *28:*568–570, 1966.
2. Birnholz J.C. and Frigoletto, F.D. Antenatal treatment of hydrocephalus. N. Engl. J. Med. *303:*1021–1023, 1981.
3. Chervenak, F.A., Ment, L.R., McClure, M., *et al.* Outcome of fetal ventriculomegaly. Lancet 2:179–181, 1984.
4. Chervenak, F.A., Berkowitz, R.L., Tortura, M., *et al.* The management of fetal hydrocephalus. Am. J. Obstet. Gynecol. *151:*933–942, 1985.
5. Clewell, W.H., Johnson, M.L., Meier, P.R., *et al.*A surgical approach to the treatment of hydrocephalus. N. Engl. J. Med. *306:*1320–1325, 1982.
6. Cochrane, D.D., Myles, S.T., Nimrod, C., *et al.* Intrauterine hydrocephalus and ventriculomegaly: associated anomalies and fetal outcome. Can. J. Neurol. Sci. *12:*51–59, 1984.
7. Fiske, C.E., Filly, R.A., and Callen, P.W. Sonographic measurement of lateral ventricular width in early ventricular dilatation. J. C. U. 9:903–907, 1981.
8. Fiske, C.E. and Filly, R.A. Ultrasound evaluation of the normal and abnormal fetal neural axis. Radiol. Clin. North Am. 20:285–296, 1982.
9. Frigoletto, F.D., Birnholz, J.C., and Greene, M.F. Antenatal treatment of hydrocephalus by ventriculoamniotic shunting. N. Engl. J. Med. 248:2496–2497, 1982.
10. Glickman, P.L., Harrison, M.R., Nakayama, D.K., *et al.* Management of ventriculomegaly in the fetus. J. Pediatr. *105:*97–108, 1984.
11. Glick, P.L., Harrison, M.R., Halks-Miller, M., *et al.* Correction of congenital hydrocephalus in utero II: efficacy of in utero shunting. J. Pediatr. Surg. *19:*870–881, 1984.
12. Harrison, M.R., Filly, R.A., Golbus, M.S., *et al.* Fetal treatment 1982. N. Engl. J. Med. *307:*1651–1652, 1982.
13. Hudgins, R.J., Edwards, M.S.B., Goldstein, R., *et al.* Natural history of fetal ventriculomegaly. Pediatrics (in press).
14. Kellner, K.R., Cruz, A.C., Gelman, S.R. *et al.* Percutaneous fetal ventriculography. J. Reprod. Med. 24:225–228, 1980.
15. Manning, F.A., Harrison, M.R., and Rodeck, C. Catheter shunts for fetal hydronephrosis and hydrocephalus. N. Engl. J. Med. *315:*336–340, 1986.
16. McCullough, D.C. and Balzer-Martin, C.A. Current prognosis in overt neonatal hydrocephalus. J. Neurosurg. 57:378–383, 1982.
17. Michejda, M. and Hodgen, G.D. In utero diagnosis and treatment of nonhuman primate fetal skeletal abnormalities I. Hydrocephalus. J.A.M.A. 246:1093–1097, 1981.
18. Miller, P., Grunstein, G., Gogol, G., *et al.* Accidental intrauterine ventriculography during termination of mid trimester pregnancy by boero technique. Neuroradiology 7:283–285, 1974.

19. Nyberg, D.A., Mack, L.A., Hirsch, J., *et al.* Fetal hydrocephalus: sonographic detection and clincal significance of associated abnormalities Radiology *163*:187–191, 1987.

20. Pretorius, D.H., Davis, K., Manco-Johnson, M.L., *et al.* Clinical course of fetal hydrocephalus: 40 cases Am. J. Radio. *144*:827–831, 1985.

21. Robertson, C.H., Lund, R.R., Soroosh, F., *et al.* Percutaneous fetal ventriculomegaly. Obstet. Gynecol. *34*:841–846, 1969.

22. Serlo, W., Kirkinen, P., Jouppila, P., *et al.* Prognostic signs in fetal hydrocephalus. Child's Nerv. Syst. *2*:93–97, 1986.

23. Venes, J.L. Management of intrauterine hydrocephalus (letter). J. Neurosurg. *58*:793–794, 1983.

24. Wright, C.H. Ultrasound in gynaecological diagnosis. In: *Gynaecological Radiology,* edited by G.H. Whitehouse, pp. 224–225, Oxford, Blackwell Scientific Publications, 1981.

CHAPTER 10

The Normal Pressure Hydrocephalus Syndrome

PETER McL. BLACK, M.D., PH.D.

INTRODUCTION

The normal pressure hydrocephalus (NPH) syndrome is a clinical syndrome of memory loss, gait disorder, urinary incontinence, and general slowing of activity. It can follow subarachnoid hemorrhage (5), trauma (3), meningitis and intracerebral surgery, and can be associated with spinal or cerebral tumors, aqueductal stenosis and Paget's disease. The most difficult cases have no known cause and are therefore idiopathic. They may be confused with Alzheimer's or Parkinson's disease. Several tests have been proposed to define the pathophysiology of this enigmatic condition, but none has yet been unequivocally successful.

Part of the present confusion reflects the syndrome's history. Psychomotor slowing and memory loss with normal cerebrospinal fluid (CSF) pressure and ventricular enlargement after subarachnoid hemorrhage were shown by Foltz and Ward (15) to be helped by shunting. It subsequently became well accepted that such a syndrome could follow particular brain insults such as surgery and subarachnoid hemorrhage. In 1964, Hakim (16) proposed that the same clinical picture might be helped by CSF diversion in patients without a known cause of hydrocephalus. Initially, this and similar reports exhibited great enthusiasm for shunting to treat memory loss in patients with large ventricles (1). Disappointing results led to a reevaluation of this policy (4, 29), with a prolonged assessment of radiological, physiological, and biochemical tests that might define the syndrome and predict the results of shunt placement. One result has been an increasing emphasis on gait disorder as a predictor of good shunt response. These attempts have been confounded by two problems: the relative rarity of the condition, and the non-physiological nature of current shunt systems. The former problem makes large series difficult to collect and evaluate; the latter leads to confusion between the results of shunting and the condition itself. Failure to improve may be a result of inadequate shunting rather than misdiagnosis of the syndrome (15). More recently, encouraging results have again been reported if strict criteria are followed (7, 25).

NORMAL PRESSURE HYDROCEPHALUS WITH KNOWN CAUSE

Pathophysiology

Most NPH cases with known cause occur when the CSF outflow is obstructed in the subarachnoid space or the ventricular system. Subarachnoid hemorrhage, meningitis, bleeding during surgery, and subdural hematomas fall into this category, causing blockade of the basal cisterns or convexity CSF pathways. Intraventricular blockade of CSF flow is caused by a second group of pathologies, including third ventricular and foramen of Monro tumors, ependymitis, and aqueductal stenosis. In children, partial obstruction of the outlets to the fourth ventricle may cause a similar pattern. In these conditions, the impetus for ventricular enlargement appears to be an increase in the resistance to CSF outflow and therefore perhaps in the pulse pressure within the ventricular system.

Diagnosis

The diagnosis of NPH is fairly straightforward if there is a history of previous trauma, subarachnoid hemorrhage, or other known predisposing condition. There is gait difficulty, which has been called gait apraxia, usually characterized by a short-stepped, wide-based gait. Recent sophisticated bioengineering studies suggest that the problem includes increased activity in extensor muscles of the arms and the legs (27). There is usually memory loss for recent memory accompanied by a general dulling of intellectual activity. Urinary incontinence is common; fecal incontinence is very rare. Although the pathophysiology of these symptoms is not clear, it appears that stretching of periventricular fibers may be important.

The results of shunting suggest that about 80% of patients with known cause will be significantly improved by placement of a ventriculoperitoneal shunt. Complications of shunt placement and their management are discussed below.

NPH in Children

The existence of NPH in children is debated. A mild learning disability or mild spastic paraparesis may be the only symptoms of such a condition, and the clinical problem may be shrugged off as "arrested hydrocephalus" (24). The author's belief is that ventricular enlargement in children may be symptomatic more often than is now suspected, but may have very subtle manifestations.

IDIOPATHIC NPH

NPH without known cause is one of the more difficult neurosurgical conditions to diagnose and treat properly. It is most common in patients over the age of 60. Its pathophysiology is unknown (18). The reason that the CSF pressure does not increase despite enlarged ventricles may be the yielding nature of parenchyma in older patients or changes in the subtle gradients that drive the ventricular enlargement (7). One experimental indicator of the latter has been the transmantle gradient which has been shown to increase in the production of experimental NPH without a rise in mean CSF pressure (11, 14, 19). A striking component of its pathophysiology in humans that has yet to be accounted for is the high prevalence of atherosclerotic disease of the cerebral arterioles and veins. Changes in cerebral blood flow (23) and in CSF neurochemistry (2) may also be partly responsible for symptomatology, but the relation of these changes to NPH remain unclear.

CLINICAL DIAGNOSIS

The hallmark of NPH of any cause remains the clinical presentation.

The gait disturbance characterizes itself by a slow, shuffling, broadbased gait. Those cases that respond best to shunting appear to have the most prominent gait disturbance. Spelberg-Sorensen et al. (27) have analyzed the gait disorder as a problem of excessive anti-gravity muscle activity, which prevents smooth organization of walking. Also characteristic is a *loss of recent memory* with a general slowing of thought processes and activity. This is not as global as the memory loss in Alzheimer's disease and is not accompanied by apraxia or visual loss. *Urinary incontinence* is accompanied by poor realization of the need to void and virtually never progresses to fecal incontinence.

The most useful diagnostic tests are lumbar puncture, computerized tomography (CT), and magnetic resonance imaging (MRI). By definition, the lumbar puncture pressure should be less than 180 mm H_2O but can, with long-term recording, be higher than this. The NPH syndrome can accompany CSF pressures greater than 180 mm H_2O, supporting the concept of a continuum of clinical symptomatology with differing CSF pressures.

CT is the most available method of assessing ventricular size. Typically NPH shows ventricular enlargement, with only modest enlargement of the subarachnoid space (13, 21). However, it has become clear recently that some degree of cerebral atrophy is quite compatible with a good response to shunting (7, 22, 26). A particularly useful finding on CT scan is periventricular low density, which appear to suggest accumulation of fluid across the ependymal lining. It does not imply CSF absorption across the ventricles but rather a kind of forcing of CSF into the parenchyma.

MRI is an important adjunct to CT scanning, especially to evaluate the possibility of diffuse parenchymal abnormality, which may lead to ventricular enlargement *ex vacuo*. It is also likely that CSF flow changes will be able to be imaged, but at the present time there has not been large-scale verification of this as a useful technique.

Isotope cisternography is still used in some centers as an indicator of CSF flow. When the pattern shows delayed ventricular emptying and little flow over the convexities, the chances are increased that shunting will be a useful maneuver; conversely, with an entirely normal cisternogram there is only very small chance of improvement with shunting.

Special Tests

The two tests which seem most important in further evaluation of idiopathic NPH are CSF dynamic testing and cerebral blood flow testing. Testing of CSF dynamics involves three possible maneuvers. The first is prolonged pressure recording, including at least 1 overnight period. This can be done either with a ventricular catheter or a lumbar catheter, or possibly with an epidural transducer. It has been shown that some patients will have increased CSF pressure during the night (13, 28). These patients tend to respond well to shunting.

Lumbar infusion testing was described by Hussey et al. (20) as a useful test; however, it appears that a number of technical and interpretative problems have made it less uniformly helpful in predicting a response to shunting than earlier studies would suggest.

Most recently, Borgesen et al. (8–10) have published extensively on evaluating NPH and predicting the response to shunting. They recommend lumboventricular perfusion as a technique. A ventricular catheter is placed for overnight recording, and the next morning a lumbar puncture is done with an 18-guage needle. Sterile lactated Ringer's is infused at a specific rate and the height of the outflow cannula is adjusted to change the perfusion pressure. Using a hypothesized CSF formation rate of 0.4 ml/min, the conductance can be calculated as the slope of the relationship between pressure and volume. The resistance is the reciprocal of the conductance. These investigators concluded that an outflow resistance greater than 12.5 ml/min/mm Hg was always accompanied by a poor shunt response. Based on their data, a paradigm for decisions about whether to proceed with shunting can be established and is presented in Figure 10.1. Their present claim is that this paradigm results in 80% shunt success even in idiopathic cases (10); without it, the success rate is approximately 65% (25).

A useful test has been to withdraw CSF by repetitive lumbar puncture, thereby causing enough continued leakage from the lumbar theca to act as a temporary shunt (29). If such maneuvers improve walking, a good result from shunting is likely. Although some neuropeptides, including somatostatin and vasopressin, may be elevated in NPH, these have not yet been linked to pathophysiology or shunt outcome (2). Like many other tests, cerebral blood flow and metabolism assessments have been thought to be helpful in NPH (23); more data are needed to establish their predictive value.

THE DECISION TO SHUNT

The decision to place a ventriculoperitoneal (VP) shunt in a patient with the NPH syndrome is not always easy. When the course of NPH is known, the clinical syndrome plus the positive history and CT findings of hydrocephalus are enough to warrant shunt placement. This decision, however, must be tempered by considerations of the patient's overall clinical condition. For patients with severe head trauma or devastating subarachnoid hemorrhage, for example, hydrocephalus and the NPH syndrome may be only one part of the overall pathological process, and shunt placement may not help.

Following subarachnoid hemorrhage there is ventricular enlargement in about two-thirds of patients, but only 10% to 15% will require shunt placement (5). Shunting is carried out early in the acute stage of ventricular dilatation if there is rapid clinical deterioration; alternatively, the NPH syndrome may occur many months after the hemorrhage. Sequential scans should be done to ascertain that progressive ventricular enlargement is not occurring in the patient with a possible NPH syndrome.

After trauma, hydrocephalus may be a result of subarachnoid block or parenchymal loss (3). In the latter it is unlikely that shunting will help, but there is no known way at present to make that distinction.

After meningitis, ventriculostomy should be used to treat symptomatic ventricular enlargement until the CSF is clear; in cases of fungal meningitis, the development of the NPH syndrome may require shunting before the CSF is sterilized. With intracranial tumors, even the removal of the tumor may not prevent the syndrome; again, close watch must be kept postoperatively with CT scanning if the patient deteriorates.

For patients with idiopathic NPH the decision is more complicated. Overall, the improvement rate is approximately 65% using clinical criteria; the likelihood of complications

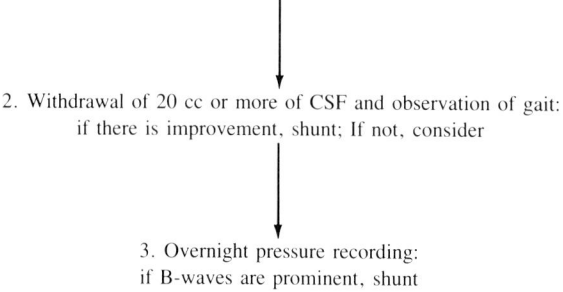

Dementia plus gait disturbance plus urinary incontinence and large ventricles
OR
Gait disturbance along in conjunction with large ventricles suggests:
1. Lumbar puncture:
If the pressure is over 180 mm H₂O, a shunt may reasonably be done without further testing; if the pressure is under 180 mm H₂O, proceed with

2. Withdrawal of 20 cc or more of CSF and observation of gait:
if there is improvement, shunt; If not, consider

3. Overnight pressure recording:
if B-waves are prominent, shunt
OR
4. Lumbar infusion or perfusion:
if resistance is greater than 12.5 ml/mins/mmHg, shunt
5. Indium or metrizamide CSF flow study:
if there is no ventricular entry, shunt

After shunting:
1. Repeat lumbar puncture or other intracranial pressure measurement to be certain that pressure has been lowered.
2. Repeat computed tomography in about 3 months to assess ventricular size and relate it to clinical improvement; if there has been no improvement and the ventricles remain large, consider placing a lower-pressure valve.

Figure 10.1. Paradigm for decision-making in idiopathic normal pressure hydrocephalus. (From, P. McL. Black and R.G. Ojemann. Cerebrospinal fluid shunts for dementia, gait disturbance, and incontinence. Clin. Neurosurg. *32*:632–656, 1985.)

is approximately 20% to 30% (7, 22, 25, 29). Factors such as the disposition of the patient to home or to a nursing home, the risks of general anesthesia, and the potential for substantial improvement must be considered.

It would appear that CT atrophy and cisternographic pattern are not particularly helpful in deciding whether to shunt a patient with the idiopathic syndrome. The prominence of gait disturbance and periventricular low absorption after CT scanning are important predictors of shunt success, however, and improvement after lumbar puncture is also helpful. Lack of improvement after lumbar puncture does not preclude a good response to shunting, however.

Many investigators now decide whether a shunt should be placed based upon a combination of clinical pattern and CT. If gait problems are prominent, they are reluctant to shunt; if the CT shows periventricular low absorption, they are more willing to do so.

Recently the author has used an implanted telesensor with ventricular catheter to monitor CSF pressure over several weeks: this system can also be used in line with a shunt to allow non-invasive monitoring (12).

SHUNT PROCEDURES

At present ventriculoperitoneal shunting is the management of choice for patients with NPH of any type. No shunt is ideal and, especially in older patients, matching the shunt system to the patient's pressure and dynamics may be difficult. Either a frontal or parieto-occipital burr hole can be used. For the frontal catheter, best landmarks for placement are 10 cm behind the nasion and 3 cm to the right of midline, with the angle of the catheter directed at the medial canthus of the ipsilateral eye and 2 cm in front of the tragus. If an occipito-parietal burr hole is used, it should be placed 6 cm above the inion and 3 cm to the right of midline. The catheter should be directed at the nasion. Meticulous preparation of the skin and minimal handling of the shunt tubing after all incisions are crucial to avoid infection.

In the abdomen, one of several sites can be used for catheter insertion. The author prefers an epigastric midline incision, which avoids the problem of dissecting through successive layers of muscle; however, the relatively thick properitoneal fat in this area occasionally makes the dissection difficult; the surgeon must be certain that the peritoneal cavity has been entered. If a subcostal or right lower quadrant incision is used, the possibility of an incisional hernia is slightly greater; in either case, the fascia over the abdominal contents must be sutured. It is important to ascertain distal flow before insertion of the peritoneal catheter.

Several different shunts are available. Typical designs use either a slit valve, whose pressure depends on the resistance to opening of slits in silastic tubing, a spring-loaded valve, which may show artifact on MRI, or a resistance valve in the peritoneal tubing, in which the outflow resistance is the important feature. These different designs have different implications for care, and it is not now possible to make a specific recommendation about the best shunt to use. It is important, though, that the surgeon be familiar with the valve design being used.

Potentially helpful adjuncts to shunting include the anti-siphon device (which prevents intra-ventricular pressure from becoming lower than the atmospheric pressure at the level of the anti-siphon device placement); a device to permit turning the shunt on or off, and various valve pressures, which the author believes should be verified by standardized technique before they are actually inserted. Valves of variable pressure may be useful in the future to 'tune' intracranial pressures in NPH patients who have shunts.

An alternative to VP shunting is ventriculoatrial (VA) shunting, which is a satisfactory but less widely used technique. The distal catheter is threaded into the common facial vein to end at the junction of the superior vena cava with the right atrium. Catheter tip localization may be confirmed by intraoperative x-ray or by electrocardiogram localization via saline electrode bridge through the atrial catheter itself. It does not appear that the prevalence of siphoning is less in the VA than in the VP shunt, or that the VA shunt is more effective than a VP shunt for treating NPH. Lumboperitoneal shunting may also be used if there is communicating hydrocephalus. The author has found that it is sometimes difficult to maintain flow in the lumboperitoneal shunt system over many years, however.

RESULTS AND COMPLICATIONS

For hydrocephalus with known cause, the results of shunting are an approximately 80% improvement in gait, mentation, and incontinence (10). In idiopathic cases, the results are less striking, with an overall improvement rate of 60% to 74% and a striking improvement in approximately 33% of patients (25). The reason for the lack of improvement is unclear, but may have to do with the length of the problem preoperatively, the nature of the disorder, or the inadequacy of available shunt systems.

Major complications of shunt placement include complications of surgery generally and those peculiar to shunt placement itself. Major surgical risks include myocardial infarction, stroke, and acute subdural hematomas (7). These occur in 17 to 32% of patients and are largely a problem for elderly and frail patients.

Other problems involve shunt placement itself. Most are related to over- or under-drainage of CSF. Over-drainage is characterized by the development of subdural collections that are usually CSF but which may have very high protein. These may result from repeated small subdural hemorrhages or a poorly understood primary problem with effusion in the region of the arachnoid membrane. Many of these can be watched, and will either remain stable or resolve with time. If these collections increase in volume, however, the appropriate management is drainage of the subdural fluid with ligation of the shunt until the collection disappears. It is not unusual for the hydrocephalus symptoms to worsen in this time, but usually 2 to 3 months are needed before the collection can be considered effectively treated and to consider re-opening the shunt. At the time of re-opening, a higher pressure valve—possibly with an anti-siphon or on-off device as well—should be considered. Alternatively, the collections themselves may be drained with a valveless shunt to the peritoneum or tied into the tubing distal to the valve by a Y connector.

Under-drainage is more subtle but perhaps as difficult to manage as over-drainage (17). In this situation the ventricles do not diminish in size despite the placement of a shunt. Symptoms persist, and the question is whether these could be ameliorated by lowering the valve pressure. There is some controversy on this matter; some authors suggest that lowering the pressure will, in fact, make a significant difference in the management of these patients (6, 7).

Other complications of shunt placement include infection and intracranial cerebral hemorrhage, both in the range of 1% to 2% in adult patients.

SUMMARY

The normal pressure hydrocephalus syndrome is an important clinical syndrome characterized by memory and gait difficulty, psychomotor slowing, and urinary incontinence. When it has a known cause, it can be improved by shunt placement in most patients. When the syndrome is of unknown etiology, the results are less striking, but still dramatic enough in some cases to warrant continued search for better criteria for shunting.

REFERENCES

1. Adams, R.D., Fisher, C.M., Hakim, S., et al. Symptomatic occult hydrocephalus with "normal" cerebrospinal fluid pressure. A treatable syndrome. N. Engl. J. Med. 273:117–126, 1965.
2. Beal, M.F., Growdon, J.H., Mazurek, M.F., et al. Cerebrospinal fluid somatostatin-like immunoreactivity in dementia. Neurology 36:294–297, 1986.
3. Beyerl, B. and Black, P.McL. Post traumatic hydrocephalus. Neurosurgery 15:257–262, 1984.
4. Black, P.McL. Idiopathic normal-pressure hydrocephalus. Results of shunting in 62 patients. J. Neurosurg. 53:371–377, 1980.
5. Black, P.McL. Hydrocephalus and vasospasm following subarachnoid hemorrhage from ruptured intracranial aneurysms. Neurosurgery 18:12–16, 1986.
6. Black, P.McL. and Ojemann RG. Hydrocephalus in adults. In Youmans JR (ed): Neurological Surgery, 3d ed. edited by J.R. Youmans, Philadelphia, W.B. Saunders, 1989, in press.
7. Black, P.McL., Ojemann, R.G., and Tzouras, A. Cerebrospinal fluid shunts for dementia, gait disturbance, and incontinence. Clin. Neurosurg. 32:632–656, 1985.
8. Borgesen, S.E. Conductance to outflow of cerebrospinal fluid in normal pressure hydrocephalus. Acta Neurochir. 71:55–62, 1985.
9. Borgesen, S.E. and Gjerris, F. Conductance to outflow of cerebrospinal fluid in normal pressure hydrocephalus. Acta Neurochir. 71:1–45, 1984.
10. Borgesen, S.E. and Gjerris, F. The predictive value of conductance to outflow of cerebrospinal fluid in normal pressure hydrocephalus. 105:65–86, 1982.
11. Conner, E.S., Black, P.McL., and Foley, L. Experimental normal pressure hydrocephalus is accompanied by increased transmantle pressure. J. Neurosurg. 61:322–328, 1984.
12. Cosman, E.R., Zervas, N.T., Chapman, P.H., et al. A telemetric pressure sensor for ventricular shunt systems. Surg. Neurol. 11:287–294, 1979.
13. Crockard, H.A., Hanlon, K., Duda, E.E., et al. Hydrocephalus as a cause of dementia: evaluation by computerized tomography and intracranial pressure monitoring. J. Neurol. Psych. 40:736–740, 1977.
14. Fishman, R.A. Occult hydrocephalus (letter). N. Engl. J. Med. 27:466–467, 1966.
15. Foltz, E.L. and Ward, A.A. Jr. Communicating hydrocephalus from subarachnoid bleeding. J. Neurosurg. 13:546–566, 1956.
16. Hakim, S. Some observations on cerebrospinal fluid pressure hydrocephalic syndrome in adults with "normal" cerebrospinal fluid pressure (recognition of a new syndrome). Thesis No. 957, Universidad Javerlana School of Medicine, Bogota, Columbia, 1964 (English translation).
17. Hakim, S. Hydraulic and mechanical mis-matching of valve shunts used in the treatment of hydrocephalus: the need for a servo-valve shunt. Devel. Med. Child. Neurol. 15:646–653, 1973.
18. Hakim, S., Venegas, J.G., and Burton, J.D. The physics of the cranial cavity, hydrocephalus, and normal pressure hydrocephalus: mechanical interpretation and mathematical model. Surg. Neurol. 5:187–210, 1976.
19. Hoff, J. and Barber, R. Transcerebral mantle pressure in normal pressure hydrocephalus. Arch. Neurol. 31:101–105, 1974.
20. Hussey, F., Schanzer, B., and Katzman, R. A simple constant infusion manometric test for measurement of cerebrospinal fluid absorption. II. Clinical studies. Neurology 20:665–680, 1970.
21. Jacobs, L. and Kinkel, W. Computerized axial transverse tomography in normal pressure hydrocephalus. Neurology 26:501–507, 1976.
22. Laws, E.R. Jr. and Mokri, B. Occult hydrocephalus: results of shunting correlated with diagnostic tests. Clin. Neurosurg. 24:316–333, 1977.
23. Meyer, J.S., Kitagaura, Y., Tanabashi, N., et al. Evaluation of treatment of normal pressure hydrocephalus—preliminary observations. Surg. Neurol. 23:121–133, 1985.
24. Milhorat, J.H. Pediatric Neurosurgery, pp. 110–112, Philadelphia, F.A. Davis, 1978.
25. Petersen, R.C., Mokri, B., and Laws, E.R. Jr. Response to shunting procedure in idiopathic normal pressure hydrocephalus. Ann. Neurol. 12:99, 1982.
26. Salmon, J.H. and Armitage, T.L. Surgical treatment of hydrocephalus ex-vacuo: ventriculo-atrial shunt for degenerative brain disease. Neurology 18:1223–1226, 1968.
27. Spelberg-Sorensen, P., Jansen, E.L., and Gjerris, F. Motor disturbance in normal-pressure hydrocephalus. Special reference to stance and gait. Arch. Neurol. 43:34–38, 1986.
28. Symon, L. and Dorsch, N.W.C. Use of long-term intracranial pressure measurement to assess hydrocephalic patients prior to shunt surgery. J. Neurosurg. 42:258–273, 1975.
29. Wood, J.H., Bartlet, D., James, A.E., Jr., et al. Normal pressure hydrocephalus. Neurology 23:706–713, 1973.

CHAPTER 11

Preventing and Treating Shunt Complications

R. MICHAEL SCOTT, M.D.

INTRODUCTION

Although shunt complications are a frequent problem on pediatric neurosurgical services, consuming much time and effort, research on prevention and treatment strategies is not as plentiful as one would wish. Consultation with experienced colleagues and empirical observation must inevitably fill the gap. The following, then, represents the author's thoughts about some common and uncommon shunt complications, along with suggestions for their treatment and prevention in pediatric patients.

VENTRICULAR CATHETER OBSTRUCTIONS

Proximal shunt obstruction is by far the most common cause of shunt complications on most neurosurgical services (8). The ventricular catheter can be blocked by adherent choroid plexus, by debris or blood in the ventricular system that occludes the catheter lumen, by brain tissue adherent to the catheter, or sometimes by another pathological process, such as tumor tissue growing around the catheter tip. In the author's opinion, attempts to prevent blockage by the addition of flanges, variable sized holes, or curves to the ventricular catheter may add to the hazards of revision, and do not prevent catheter occlusion.

'Stuck' Ventricular Catheter

When ventricular catheter obstruction is diagnosed during surgery, normally the catheter is removed and replaced with a new one. At times, however, the catheter may be stuck to the ventricular walls and choroid plexus. Although it is tempting to leave a stuck catheter in place, it is probably preferable to remove all non-functioning shunt apparatus at revision, since any later infection may result in colonization of retained catheters, leading to brain abscess or recurring infections. Usually, gradual traction can be applied to the catheter and the adherence to the ventricle wall will give way until the catheter can be removed. Care must be taken to remove it slowly while looking for adherent choroid plexus along the tubing as it is delivered from the burr hole; this material should be coagulated off the catheter as it is encountered and resected.

Nevertheless, attempts to remove a tightly adherent catheter may result in intraventricular bleeding, which could cause significant disability and at the very least reblock the newly inserted catheter, so occasionally the catheter must be left in place.

Intraventricular Bleeding Following Catheter Removal

When bleeding that does not stop readily occurs within the ventricle, small amounts of saline should be irrigated through a new catheter until the CSF clears; this takes considerable time and patience. If the newly placed catheter then contains any blood clot, it is prudent to change it again, if possible, before closing, lest the shunt re-occlude. If bleeding never really stops, the catheter should be converted to external drainage for bedside observation if the shunt is reconnected, the patient must be observed frequently by computerized tomography (CT) and clinically for evidence of deterioration secondary to additional intraventricular bleeding or from recurring hydrocephalus caused by more obstruction.

115

Ventricular Catheter Occlusion

This shunt complication is not easily avoided. Standard teaching dictates that the shunt tip should be placed in the frontal horn anterior to the choroid plexus, which would otherwise readily adhere to the catheter and block its openings. This is probably easiest with a catheter placed via a frontal burr hole (1), but as the ventricle shrinks following treatment of the hydrocephalus the catheter tip is brought into approximation with the choroid and ventricular walls. An occipital catheter can be placed with its tip anterior to the foramen of Monro by determining the appropriate length from the preoperative CT scan; however, when the child's head grows and the ventricle shrinks, the same process will occur. Moreover, throughout most of its length the catheter frequently will lie in apposition with the choroid.

A potentially avoidable cause of ventricular catheter occlusion is reaction to foreign material on the catheter. When ventricular catheters are examined microscopically following removal, foreign body giant cells or birefringent crystals, suture remnants, or other foreign materials occasionally can be found in the debris occluding the catheter lumen (9). This suggests that careful handling of the ventricular catheter before placement—implanting the catheter promptly following removal from its package, avoiding excessive manipulation of it, using lint-free drapes—might lessen this risk.

DISTAL SHUNT OBSTRUCTIONS

Inadequate Initial Placement

Distal occlusions of ventriculo-peritoneal shunt systems are relatively rare and are usually related to only a few causes. The catheter may be positioned poorly at the time of its initial placement, usually from instillation into the pre-peritoneal fat rather than the peritoneal cavity proper. Several clues at the time of surgery suggest that the catheter is being placed improperly: it coils or passes with some difficulty into the abdomen; cerebrospinal fluid (CSF) wells up around the peritoneal entrance site, indicating poor CSF diffusion into the peritoneal cavity. Postoperatively, the shunt x-rays will demonstrate coiling of the tubing into a tight superficial circle, and abdominal ultrasound will demonstrate increasing extra-perito-

neal CSF around the tubing. This complication will be avoided if the surgeon always uses a familiar, standard approach to the peritoneal cavity. If an unfamiliar exposure is necessitated by previous surgery or other reasons, the anatomy is often clarified by making the incision and fascial openings large enough to permit good visualization and adequate retraction; prepping and draping should always be planned with this in mind. (A headlight and magnification are also helpful.) If there are adhesions or the anatomy looks unusual, an experienced surgical colleague should be consulted. A small peritoneal opening should be gently probed with a penfield dissector to ensure that it is in free communication with the peritoneal cavity before the tubing is inserted.

Peritoneal Loculations

Distal obstruction can also be caused by low-grade shunt infections, which lead to encystment and loculations of the peritoneal contents around the catheter tip (6). That shunt infection is causing the obstruction may not be readily apparent in the absence of fever or other systemic signs. Cultures will be positive only if the most rigorous attempts are made to culture what are frequently fastidious organisms, and diagnosis may be quite difficult. The pseudocyst itself may be obvious upon palpation of the abdomen, and will be confirmed by abdominal ultrasound. Ultrasound-guided percutaneous aspiration of the peritoneal culture collections may aid in management if the patient is not acutely ill from malfunction. Appropriate treatment is discussed in Chapter 8.

Peritoneal Catheter Withdrawal

The growing pediatric patient can present with a shunt whose tip no longer sits in the peritoneal cavity. This problem is entirely preventable if adequate tubing is inserted initially. For more than a decade, the author has inserted the entire length of the 90 cm commercially available peritoneal catheters in children of all sizes and weights—with the exception of extremely small prematures weighing less than 1 kg—and bowel perforation or tube kinking has not been a problem. Nevertheless, if the surgeon feels that a shorter peritoneal catheter is appropriate, the patient should be followed by periodic x-rays of the abdomen to observe residual tubing, and an elective revision carried out when the tubing tip nears the peritoneal opening. Placing a small metal clip near the entry site helps in identifying the peritoneal opening in subsequent x-rays. When a follow-up x-ray is obtained it is helpful to measure the distance from the lower end of the cranial valve to the abdominal incision and follow this measurement yearly instead of taking frequent x-rays.

If the shunt is to be lengthened electively, it is important that this be carried out from just below the valve downward to avoid subsequent disconnection at a distally placed connector (see below).

SHUNT DISCONNECTION

Asymptomatic Disconnections

Disconnections are often obvious on palpation or on shunt x-rays, and a gap in the tubing or a soft lump at the disconnection site may be the patient's initial complaint. An asymptomatic disconnection does not mean that the shunt is non-functional. Patients with known disconnections of long duration may eventually develop symptoms of shunt obstruction, and exploration reveals fibrous tracts around the shunt system that are capable of conveying CSF past the area of tube disruption to the distal tubing. Patients and families should be informed that asymptomatic disconnection is possible, and that elective reconnection should be considered if CT scanning shows small ventricles or there is a history of shunt dependence.

Preventing Disconnections

Disconnections may be caused by assembly errors in the initial shunt system. Shunt tubing frequently disconnects at stress points where connectors rub against silastic tubing, fraying and finally breaking it. For example, connectors should not be placed low in the neck adjacent to bulky valves, where neck movements could easily fatigue and tear the tubing. All connections should be tightly secured with 2-0 non-absorbable suture that does not cut through the tubing and resists disconnection when it is tugged firmly as a strength test before closure.

A common cause of shunt disconnection is the improper use of connectors distal to the valve apparatus. Because a soft-tissue reaction will occur around suture material and metal or nylon connectors, as the patient grows the connector complex will not move through the subcutaneous tissues as easily as the silastic tubing

itself, and the shunt apparatus becomes bound at these sites. With continued growth, the tubing is stretched because of its subcutaneous binding and it will break eventually. Some shunt systems unfortunately have a built-in propensity for this complication, particularly if the shunt valve has a relatively long distal limb with an attached connector. At follow-up children with these systems who have grown are often observed to have tubing in the anterior cervical region that is taut and stretched.

To avoid repeated disconnections, therefore, the author recommends that distal revisions of peritoneal shunts in the growing patient involve replacing the entire tubing just distal to the cranial valve, rather than lengthening it at the peritoneum entrance and placing a connector there.

Tubing may rupture secondary to trauma, a phenomenon more likely the longer a shunt is in position. As the tubing ages, calcific deposits build up around it or the tubing wall itself degenerates, making cracking or tearing with minor trauma more likely. Occasionally, the tubing will kink and occlude even without trauma, and surgeons will probably notice such occlusion more frequently as their patients age. Firm tubular accretions can be palpated over the tubing, particularly in the upper thorax where the tubing has been relatively immobile for years. The tubing should be replaced if the area is painful, tender, or subject to irritation or trauma because of its location (particularly over the clavicle). The tubing can be so bound into the soft tissues that multiple incisions may be necessary to remove it.

Shunt Migration

The shunt apparatus can also dislodge and migrate, and the author has seen patients in whom the entire shunt apparatus, including valve and distal tubing, has migrated into the ventricle or distally into the neck or abdomen. (These cases are unusual; the child in whom the apparatus migrated into the ventricle, for example, had a huge head permitting this complication to occur gradually without detection.) Nevertheless, lesser degrees of dislocation can occur depending on the shunt's bulk, the length of time it is in place (in time, scarring around valves and reservoirs tends to prevent dislodgment), and redundancy of subcutaneous tissue planes that permit the tubing to slide out of its original position. This complication can be avoided upon insertion by securing the shunt proximally directly to the pericranium. Distal connectors, which later can cause traction on the more proximal apparatus (leading to its dislocation), should not be used.

PREVENTING SHUNT INFECTIONS

Infections are a common complication of ventricular shunting, (see Chapter 8). Although many shunt infections are probably not preventable, some measures probably help to reduce the risk of infection related to inoculation at the time of surgery. Choux of Marseille (3), for example, has succeeded in preventing infection completely in a series of 274 shunt operations. His regimen involves the minimal handling of the shunt apparatus by an experienced two-person surgical team without a scrub nurse, the use of high-dose intravenous antibiotics before the procedure (100 mg/kg of oxacillin), and the scheduling of all shunts and shunt revisions early in the day before other scheduled procedures. Although many North American neurosurgeons cannot arrange their surgical schedules this way, if long procedures and heavy operating room traffic potentiate contamination, adapting Choux's protocol makes sense. The author agrees that limiting scrub personnel, shunt exposure and handling, and operating time are important, as is using only experienced personnel. Prophylactic antibiotics should probably be used at the time of shunt surgery, although the literature does not yet unquestionably confirm their benefit. It must also be acknowledged that many shunt infections are unrelated to inoculation during surgery, but occur following transient bacteremias or because of age-related lowered immunological competence or other poorly understood factors. The very high prevalence of shunt infection in premature infants is a common observation, for example (10).

SEIZURE DISORDERS

Seizures may occur following ventricular shunting. The prevalence of this condition has been variably reported from 5% to 48% (5, 7), and it has been suggested that the choice of burr-hole site is a contributing factor, with a higher risk of seizures occurring in frontal rather than occipital burr holes (4). This report has not been confirmed subsequently (12), and the author believes that burr-hole location is not significant in the etiology of postoperative seizures. The author has observed, however, that shunt infection resulting in ventriculitis does increase the risk of seizures in the myelomeningocele population (2), indicating the importance of aggressively treating shunt infection in any patient. It should also be noted that seizures may occasionally signal the onset of shunt malfunction in the susceptible patient (perhaps related to stretching of cortex and displacement of the ventricular catheter with increasing intraventricular pressure), and should not always be dismissed as being unrelated to shunt function. Prophylactic seizure medications are not indicated for routine management, however.

EXTRACEREBRAL CSF COLLECTIONS

Symptomatic extracerebral CSF collections are a dreaded complication. This phenomenon is particularly likely in the patient with very large ventricles and/or calvarium, and it is a major concern in the delayed treatment of patients with congenital hydrocephalus or of any symptomatic hydrocephalic patient with considerable atrophy. Although some small and asymptomatic CSF accumulations following shunting require no treatment, it is necessary for those that cause headache or neurological deficit. CSF drainage by burr hole alone is rarely effective, since so much of the accumulation is passively induced and tends to recur. If there has been some bleeding or the CSF is under pressure, however, simple drainage may suffice to obtain symptomatic relief. The obvious pressure differential between the subdural and intraventricular compartments tends to perpetuate these collections, and definitive treatment should be directed toward increasing the intraventricular pressure relative to that in the subdural space. Valve pressures alone make little real difference in the erect patient's intraventricular pressure, and revising the shunt valve to a higher pressure often does not significantly raise it. Temporary ligation of the shunt system with burr-hole drainage is another possible solution that frequently works, but it requires reopening the shunt, which occasionally may cause the hygroma to recur; this technique cannot be used in a shunt-dependent patient. An ingenious method to ligate and then 'reopen' the shunt with only one procedure in a patient who is not shunt-dependent is to ligate the shunt with a chromic suture; the suture gradually disintegrates, allowing the shunt to spontaneously reopen. In certain patients, an on-off valve can be used to turn the shunt off for as long as the patient tolerates it after the hygroma is drained, or to periodically open and close the shunt to prevent hygroma recurrence. The author does not routinely use these valves because occasionally they can be turned off inadvertently, and their bulky configuration makes placement in children difficult. Large hygromas can be treated by shunting to the peritoneum, a technique especially attractive in the shunt-dependent patient. The existing shunt system can be used for this procedure by placing a burr hole over the hygroma into which a short catheter for drainage can be placed. This catheter in turn can be connected into the existing shunt system below the valve assembly to ensure that the pressure in the subdural space is lower than the valve-influenced intraventricular pressure. Bilateral subdural hygromas are almost always contiguous and can be drained by a single catheter.

PNEUMOCEPHALUS

Spontaneous pneumocephalus following ventricular shunting can be extraordinarily difficult to treat. These patients fall into 2 categories—those shunted for post-traumatic hydrocephalus, and those shunted for congenital hydrocephalus. In the first group, skull-base fractures permitted ingress of air once intracranial pressure (ICP) has been lowered by the shunt. In the second group, the hydrocephalus has created a sustained increase in ICP over time (9), resulting in a thinning of the skull base and enlargement of congenital bone defects. When the shunt is finally placed, air enters through these bone and dural defects formerly tamponaded by brain under pressure. These patients are difficult to treat, particularly if they have become shunt-dependent, since the site of air ingress is often unusually located and there is no obvious CSF leak because of the functioning shunt. If the shunt is externalized and placed on variable pressure drainage, manipulating ICP (with the aid of the usual diagnostic measures such as radioisotope tracer studies and CT studies of skull base augmented by intrathecal contrast) may show a CSF leak site. The skull defect can then be repaired. In shunt-dependent patients with congenital aqueduct occlusion, the ICP can never be raised enough to indicate the leak, and the congenital bony abnormalities are often too small to detect by the usual studies. One such patient of the author's underwent 2 anterior fossa explorations before an astute radiologist detected a defect in the sphenoid, repair of which (using trans-ethmoidal approach) finally stopped air from entering the cranium.

OVER-DRAINAGE SYNDROME

This syndrome is usually seen in children shunted early in life, although it also can be seen in adults treated for hydrocephalus from various causes. The patient presents with headache or dizziness that typically depend upon position—worse when erect, better when prone. The CT scan may show small or slit ventricles, but the syndrome should not be confused with the high-pressure ''slit ventricle syndrome.'' The shunt reservoir usually can be aspirated easily, and a low ICP is usually obtained. Patients may need revision because of disabling symptoms, although the syndrome might only be transient following the initial shunt placement. The simplest and most effective revision technique is to upgrade the valve to a higher pressure system, since only 20 mm to 30 mm of water additional valve pressure is often enough to relieve symptoms. Rarely, an anti-siphon device is needed, but the author does not use this equipment primarily because it tends to malfunction with time.

BOWEL PERFORATION

Rarely, the intestines may be injured when a peritoneal catheter is placed by using a trocar in a peritoneal cavity scarred from previous surgery. When opening the peritoneal cavity directly, the surgeon can mistake the intestinal wall for the peritoneum, or if a viscus is adherent to the peritoneal wall when it is incised, it may be perforated. The literature provides no clear guidelines on management, but the author believes that the bowel opening should be closed immediately with inverting sutures to approximate serosa, and that the wound and distal shunt should be considered contaminated. The shunt tubing should be externalized through a thoracic incision, and the patient observed until it is certain that both the peritoneum and shunt system are uninfected. The shunt can then be internalized elsewhere in the abdomen.

Rarely, bowel perforation occurs spontaneously some—time after shunt insertion. (With the gradual disappearance of spring-loaded peritoneal catheters, the author has not seen this problem since 1981.) This complication may be signalled by the appearance of the shunt tubing at the anus, or by symptoms of shunt infection or obstruction combined with shunt x-rays that indicate that the tubing follows the course of the colon or small intestine. The opening into the intestinal lumen is often small and self-sealing, and laparotomy is rarely required. The tubing should be divided well above the abdomen and externalized; an assistant can then pull the tubing out of the abdomen through a lower incision over the tubing or from the anus if it presents there. After a period of observation, the shunt can be re-internalized.

SLIT VENTRICLE SYNDROME

This shunt complication is discussed in detail in Chapter 7. The author has found several points to be helpful in managing this syndrome in children. Most appear to have partial obstruction of their ventricular catheters, and CT scans show definite ventricular dilatation during symptomatic periods. Often revision of the ventricular catheter alone will solve the problem. If there is any doubt that the patient has raised ICP as well as the small ventricular system, and the patient has communicating hydrocephalus, a lumbar puncture to measure ICP pressure is advisable. Occasionally, these taps are therapeutic—draining off enough CSF to normalize pressure may get the patient over a temporary ICP crisis and no further treatment will be required. Similarly, if the episodes seem clearly related to a systemic process such as a viral illness, the author has treated the syndrome with high dose dexamethasone for several days; the swelling and pressure occurring with this syndrome appear to respond particularly well to this regimen in certain children. If the problem is recurrent despite these measures, LP shunting can be carried out in patients with communicating hydrocephalus. In the patient with refractory symptoms, Wisoff and Epstein (see Chapter 7) advocate extensive cranial decompression. The author has rarely had to resort to this procedure, and recommends that before attempting it the usual measures of ventricular catheter revision, valve upgrade, and anti-siphon device placement be tried. The child should undergo a period of ICP monitoring to ensure that the diagnosis of elevated ICP is correct.

ISOLATED VENTRICLE SYNDROMES

Ventricular asymmetries commonly develop following ventricular shunting for reasons discussed in Chapter 2, and it is not uncommon to note that the ventricle with the catheter within it is smaller than its opposite. Usually, these asymmetries are asymptomatic, and surgeons should be cautious about diagnosing a trapped ventricle syndrome simply on the basis of differential ventricular size, no matter how dramatic. Before placing another catheter into the opposite ventricle and complicating later shunt management, the degree of communication should be ascertained by tapping the shunt, measuring ICP, and instilling water-soluble contrast for immediate and delayed CT studies. The author believes that symptomatic trapped lateral ventricles are rare. Magnetic resonance imaging (MRI) flow studies will shortly be able to confirm flow across intraventricular foramina.

Bona fide trapped ventricular syndromes are relatively easy to diagnose. Signs include increased ICP syndromes or neurologic deficits; in the case of trapped fourth ventricles, patients will present with headache, ataxia, lower cranial nerves signs, and dizziness and vertigo. It is important that the shunting apparatus is designed to equilibrate pressures in both supratentorial and infratentorial compartments, and the fourth ventricular catheter should be connected to the system already in place above its valve. This type of system also simplifies subsequent revisions. A frequent problem with fourth ventricular catheters is that the typical burr hole is placed too high in the suboccipital area to reach the subtentorial compartment, or too far lateral to allow the surgeon to easily estimate the length and depth of the dilated fourth ventricle. The author uses a midline approach to cannulate the fourth ventricle under direct vision, or makes a wide craniectomy to permit the use of intra-operative ultrasound.

SOME COMMON QUESTIONS

"Will my child ever be shunt-independent?" One is never really certain about the answer to this question, but the answer can be definitely "No" if the type of hydrocephalus is known to

be non-communicating (such as aqueduct occlusion) or there is a history of symptomatic shunt obstruction. In children with myelomeningoceles, the author answers in the negative even though obstructed shunts may occasionally appear to be asymptomatic in this group. Such children may be decompressing CSF into the central canal of the spinal cord, which may have harmful late sequelae; shunt dependency should therefore be assumed. In other children, the author relies on CT scanning to help answer this question. If the ventricles are very small with the shunt in place, the author assumes shunt dependency—although there must be exceptions to this rule. If the ventricular system is moderately enlarged, parents can be told that there is a possibility that the shunt might no longer be needed. Such a shunt should never be removed arbitrarily, and in fact, the author never removes even a nonfunctioning shunt unless there are important reasons to do so, for fear of causing intraventricular bleeding if the catheter is stuck.

"What are the limitations on activity of my shunted child?" The author knows of no guidelines on this question, and counsels patients to be as active as their neurologic status permits. Direct contact sports such as football are proscribed, but skating, skiing, and cycling are permitted if helmets are worn. The author believes that these patients have an increased risk of intracerebral bleeding with head trauma, but this must be balanced against normalization of as many activities as possible, an important goal. If asymptomatic subdural CSF collections are noted on routine scans, however, extra caution should probably be observed (see above).

"How often will my child need x-rays?" The author follows ventricular size of shunted newborns and children with open fontanelles by cranial ultrasound following placement of the shunt, at the first post-operative visit when it is clear that the shunt is functioning, and thereafter when indicated based on head circumference measurements and clinical indications. When the fontanelle closes, a baseline CT or MRI is obtained, and repeated at least at 5-year intervals until the patient is grown. The parents are questioned at yearly follow-up visits about school performance as well as the usual symptoms of shunt malfunction, and scans are performed earlier when clinically indicated.

REFERENCES

1. Albright, A.L., Haines, S.J., and Taylor, F.H. Function of parietal and frontal shunts in childhood hydrocephalus. J. Neurosurg. *69*:883–86, 1988.
2. Bartoshesky, L.E., Haller, J., Scott, R.M., *et al.* Seizures in children with meningomyelocele. Am. J. Dis. Child *193*:400–402, 1985.
3. Choux, M., Lena, G., Genitori, L., *et al.* Shunt implantation: toward zero infection. Child's Nerv. Syst. *4*:181, 1988.
4. Dan, N.G. and Wade, M.J. The incidence of epilepsy after ventricular shunting procedures. J. Neurosurg. *65*:19–21, 1986.
5. DiRocco, C., Iannelli, A., Pallini, R., *et al.* Epilepsy and its correlation with cerebral ventricular shunting procedures in infantile hydrocephalus. J. Pediat. Neurosci. *1*:255–263, 1985.
6. Fischer, E.G. and Shillito, J. Large abdominal cysts: a complication of peritoneal shunts. Case report. J. Neurosurg. *31*:441–444, 1969.
7. Graebner, R.W. and Celesia, G.G. EEG findings in hydrocephalus and their relation to shunting procedures. Electroencephalogr. Clin. Neurophysiol. *35*:517–521, 1973.
8. McLaurin, R.L. Ventricular shunts: Complications and results. In: *Pediatric Neurosurgery*, edited by R.L. McLaurin, L. Schut, J.L.Venes, and F. Epstein, pp. 219–229, Philadelphia, W.B. Saunders, 1989.
9. Ruge, J.R., Cerullo, L.J., and McLone, D.G. Pneumocephalus in patients with CSF shunts. J. Neurosurg. *63*:532–536, 1985.
10. Scarf, T.B., Anderson, D.E., Anderson, C.L., *et al.* Complications of ventricular-peritoneal shunts in premature infants. In: *Concepts of Pediatric Neurosurgery*, Vol. 4, edited by R.P Humphrey, pp. 81 87, Basel, Karger, 1983.
11. Sekhar, L.N., Moossy, J., and Guthkelch, A.N. Malfunctioning ventriculoperitoneal shunts. Clinical and pathological features. J. Neurosurg. *56*:411–416, 1982.
12. Venes, J.L. and Dauser, R.C. Epilepsy following ventricular shunt placement. J. Neurosurg. *66*:154–555, 1987.

Index

Page numbers in *italics* denote figures; those followed by "t" denote tables.